Learning L ....es

Implications for
Psychiatric Treatment

EDITED BY

Laurence L. Greenhill, M.D.

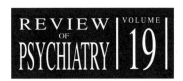

REVIEW OF PSYCHIATRY | VOLUME 19 |

No. 5

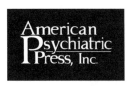

American Psychiatric Press, Inc.

Washington, DC
London, England

Note: The authors have worked to ensure that all information in this book concerning drug dosages, schedules, and routes of administration is accurate as of the time of publication and consistent with standards set by the U.S. Food and Drug Administration and the general medical community. As medical research and practice advance, however, therapeutic standards may change. For this reason and because human and mechanical errors sometimes occur, we recommend that readers follow the advice of a physician who is directly involved in their care or the care of a member of their family.

Copyright © 2000 American Psychiatric Press, Inc.
03   02   01   00   4   3   2   1

ALL RIGHTS RESERVED
Manufactured in the United States of America on acid-free paper

American Psychiatric Press, Inc.
1400 K Street, NW
Washington, DC 20005
www.appi.org

The correct citation for this book is

> Greenhill LL (ed.): *Learning Disabilities: Implications for Psychiatric Treatment* (Review of Psychiatry Series, Vol. 19, No. 5; Oldham JO and Riba MB, series eds.). Washington, DC, American Psychiatric Press, 2000

Library of Congress Cataloging-in-Publication Data
Learning disabilities : implications for psychiatric treatment / edited by
    Laurence L. Greenhill.
        p. ; cm. — (Review of psychiatry series; v. 19, no. 5)
    Includes bibliographical references and index.
    ISBN 0-88048-383-0 (alk. paper)
    1. Learning disabilities. 2. Attention-deficit hyperactivity disorders.
    I. Greenhill, Laurence L. II. Review of psychiatry series ; v. 19, 5.
        [DNLM: 1. Learning Disorders. 2. Attention Deficit Disorder with
    Hyperactivity. 3. Dyslexia. WS 110 L43752 2000]
    RC394.L37 L43 2000
    616.85´889—dc21

                                                                    00-023123

British Library Cataloguing in Publication Data
A CIP record is available from the British Library.

Review of Psychiatry Series ISSN 1041-5882

Contents

Contributors

Howard Abikoff, Ph.D.
Professor of Clinical Psychiatry, New York University Child Study Center, New York University School of Medicine, New York, New York

L. Eugene Arnold, M.D., M.Ed.
Professor Emeritus of Psychiatry, Ohio State University, Columbus, Ohio

Mark Davies, M.P.H.
Research Scientist, Department of Child Psychiatry, New York State Psychiatric Institute, New York, New York

Jack M. Fletcher, Ph.D.
Department of Pediatrics, University of Texas Medical School–Houston, Houston, Texas

Steve Forness, Ed.D.
Professor, Department of Psychiatry and Biobehavioral Science, University of California Los Angeles, Los Angeles, California

Laurence L. Greenhill, M.D.
Professor of Clinical Psychiatry, New York State Psychiatric Institute, New York, New York

Frank Gresham, Ph.D.
Distinguished Professor, Department of Education, University of California, Riverside, Riverside, California

Tom Hanley, Ed.D.
Education Research Analyst, Office of Special Education Programs, U.S. Department of Education, Washington, D.C.

Lily Hechtman, M.D., F.R.C.P.C.
Professor of Psychiatry and Pediatrics and Director of Research, Division of Child Psychiatry, Montreal Children's Hospital, Montreal, Quebec, Canada

Stephen Hinshaw, Ph.D.
Professor of Psychology, Department of Clinical Psychology, University of California at Berkeley, Berkeley, California

Betsy Hoza, Ph.D.
Associate Professor, Department of Psychological Sciences, Purdue University, West Lafayette, Indiana

Rachel G. Klein, Ph.D.
Professor of Psychiatry, Child Study Center, New York University Medical Center, New York, New York

Salvatore Mannuzza, Ph.D.
Research Professor, Child Study Center, New York University Medical Center, New York, New York

Brooke Molina, Ph.D.
Assistant Professor, Department of Psychiatry, Western Psychiatric Institute and Clinic, Pittsburgh, Pennsylvania

Carol Odbert, B.S.
Statistician, Department of Health and Human Services/Public Health Service, National Institutes of Mental Health/National Institute of Health, Bethesda, Maryland

John M. Oldham, M.D.
Director, New York State Psychiatric Institute; Dollard Professor and Acting Chairman, Department of Psychiatry, Columbia University College of Physicians and Surgeons, New York, New York

Betty B. Osman, Ph.D.
Psychologist, Child and Adolescent Service, Department of Behavioral Health, White Plains Hospital Center, White Plains, New York

William Pelham, Ph.D.
Associate Professor, Department of Psychiatry and Psychology, State University of New York–Buffalo, Buffalo, New York

Kenneth R. Pugh, Ph.D.
Department of Pediatrics, Yale University School of Medicine; Haskins Laboratories, New Haven, Connecticut

Michelle B. Riba, M.D.
Clinical Associate Professor of Psychiatry and Associate Chair for Education and Academic Affairs, Department of Psychiatry, University of Michigan Health System, Ann Arbor, Michigan

Ann Schulte, Ph.D.
Associate Professor, Department of Psychology, North Carolina State University, Raleigh, North Carolina

Joanne Severe, M.S.
Chief, Biostatistics and Data Management Unit, Division of Services and Intervention Research, National Institute of Mental Health, Bethesda, Maryland

Bennett A. Shaywitz, M.D.
Departments of Pediatrics and Neurology, Yale University School of Medicine, New Haven, Connecticut

Sally E. Shaywitz, M.D.
Department of Pediatrics, Yale University School of Medicine, New Haven, Connecticut

Stephen Simpson, M.A.
Psychologist, Department of Pediatrics, University of California, Irvine, Irvine, California

James M. Swanson, Ph.D.
Professor, Department of Pediatrics, and Director, Child Development Center, University of California, Irvine, Irvine, California

Rosemary Tannock, Ph.D.
Senior Scientist, Research Institute of The Hospital for Sick Children; Associate Professor of Psychiatry, University of Toronto, Toronto, Ontario, Canada

Michael Wasdell, M.A.
Senior Data Production Coordinator, Department of Pediatrics, University of California, Irvine, Irvine, California

Karen Wells, Ph.D.
Associate Professor of Medical Psychology, Department of Psychiatry, Duke University Medical Center, Durham, North Carolina

Timothy Wigal, Ph.D.
Associate Professor, Department of Pediatrics, University of California, Irvine, Irvine, California

Introduction to the Review of Psychiatry Series

John M. Oldham, M.D.
Michelle B. Riba, M.D., Series Editors

2000 REVIEW OF PSYCHIATRY SERIES TITLES

- *Learning Disabilities: Implications for Psychiatric Treatment*
  EDITED BY LAURENCE L. GREENHILL, M.D.
- *Psychotherapy for Personality Disorders*
  EDITED BY JOHN G. GUNDERSON, M.D., AND GLEN O. GABBARD, M.D.
- *Ethnicity and Psychopharmacology*
  EDITED BY PEDRO RUIZ, M.D.
- *Complementary and Alternative Medicine and Psychiatry*
  EDITED BY PHILIP R. MUSKIN, M.D.
- *Pain: What Psychiatrists Need to Know*
  EDITED BY MARY JANE MASSIE, M.D.

The advances in knowledge in the field of psychiatry and the neurosciences in the last century can easily be described as breathtaking. As we embark on a new century and a new millennium, we felt that it would be appropriate for the 2000 Review of Psychiatry Series monographs to take stock of the state of that knowledge at the interface between normality and pathology. Although there may be nothing new under the sun, we are learning more about not-so-new things, such as how we grow and develop; who we are; how to differentiate between just being different from one another and being ill; how to recognize, treat, and perhaps prevent illness; how to identify our unique vulnerabilities; and how to deal with the inevitable stress and pain that await each of us.

In the early years of life, for example, how can we tell whether a particular child is just rowdier, less intelligent, or more adventuresome than another child—or is, instead, a child with a learning or behavior disorder? Clearly, the distinction is crucial, because newer and better treatments that now exist for early-onset disorders can smooth the path and enhance the chances for a solid future for children with such disorders. Yet, inappropriately labeling and treating a rambunctious but normal child can create problems rather than solve them. Greenhill and colleagues guide us through these waters, illustrating that a highly sophisticated methodology has been developed to make this distinction with accuracy, and that effective treatments and interventions are now at hand.

Once we have successfully navigated our way into early adulthood, we are supposed to have a pretty good idea (so the advice books say) of who we are. Of course, this stage of development does not come easy, nor at the same time, for all. Again, a challenge presents itself—that is, to differentiate between widely disparate varieties of temperament and character and when extremes of personality traits and styles should be recognized as disorders. And even when traits are so extreme that little dispute exists that a disorder is present, does that disorder represent who the person is, or is it something the individual either inherited or developed and might be able to overcome? In the fifth century B.C., Hippocrates described different personality types that he proposed were correlated with specific "body humors"; this ancient principle remains quite relevant, though the body humors of today are neurotransmitters. How low CNS serotonin levels need to be, for example, to produce disordered impulsivity is still being determined, yet new symptom-targeted treatment of such conditions with SSRIs is now well accepted. What has been at risk as the neurobiology of personality disorders has become increasingly understood is the continued recognition of the importance of psychosocial treatments for these disorders. Gunderson and Gabbard and their colleagues review the surprisingly robust evidence for the effectiveness of these approaches, including new uses and types of cognitive-behavioral and psychoeducational methods.

It is not just differences in personality that distinguish us from one another. Particularly in our new world of global communication and population migration, ethnic and cultural differences are more often part of life in our own neighborhoods than just exotic and unfamiliar aspects of faraway lands. Despite great strides overcoming fears and prejudices, much work remains to be done. At the same time, we must learn more about ways that we are different (not better or worse) genetically and biologically, because uninformed ignorance of these differences leads to unacceptable risks. Ruiz and colleagues carefully present what we now know and do not know about ethnicity and its effects on pharmacokinetics and pharmacodynamics.

An explosion of interest in and information about wellness—not just illness—surrounds us. How to achieve and sustain a healthy lifestyle, how to enhance successful aging, and how to benefit from "natural" remedies saturate the media. Ironically, although this seems to be a new phenomenon, the principles of complementary or alternative medicine are ancient. Some of our oldest and most widely used medications are derived from plants and herbs, and Eastern medicine has for centuries relied on concepts of harmony, relaxation, and meditation. Again, as the world shrinks, we are obligated to be open to ideas that may be new to us but not to others and to carefully evaluate their utility. Muskin and colleagues present a careful analysis of the most familiar and important components of complementary and alternative medicine, presenting a substantial database of information, along with tutorials on non-Western (hence nontraditional to us) concepts and beliefs.

Like it or not, life presents us with stress and pain. Pain management has not typically figured into mainstream psychiatric training or practice (with the exception of consultation-liaison psychiatry), yet it figures prominently in the lives of us all. Massie and colleagues provide us with a primer on what psychiatrists should know about the subject, and there is a great deal indeed that we should know.

Many other interfaces exist between psychiatry as a field of medicine, defining and treating psychiatric illnesses, and the rest of medicine—and between psychiatry and the many paths of the life cycle. These considerations are, we believe, among our top priorities as we begin the new millennium, and these volumes provide an in-depth review of some of the most important ones.

Foreword

Laurence L. Greenhill, M.D.

Approximately 5% of all public school students are identified as having a learning disability. Learning disability is not a single disorder, but includes disabilities in any of seven areas related to reading, language, and mathematics, including receptive language (listening), expressive language (speaking), basic reading skills, reading comprehension, written expression, mathematics calculation, and mathematical reasoning. Although the prevalence of learning disability has increased in the past 20 years, no consensus about the "real" prevalence of learning disability has been reached because no agreed-on definition of learning disability with objective criteria has been identified. As Lyon (1996) noted, the "field continues to be beset by pervasive, and occasionally contentious, disagreements about the definition of the disorder, diagnostic criteria, assessment practices, treatment procedures, and educational policies." It is into this arena that the authors of these chapters have taken their stand.

Rachel G. Klein, Ph.D., and Salvatore Mannuzza, Ph.D., examine the adult psychiatric status of children with reading disorders (n = 104) without evidence of significant psychiatric problems, referred to as *uncomplicated reading disorders*. A comparison group (n = 129) of age-matched control subjects also was followed up and evaluated. Evaluations at the 16-year follow-up were conducted with raters blind as to the knowledge of childhood history. This prospective, longitudinal, double-blind study found that children who had uncomplicated reading disorders at age 10 years, but assessed as adults, had lower IQ scores, lower educational attainment, lower occupational attainment, and more psychiatric diagnoses. Thus, learning disabilities in childhood confer a risk for a wide range of morbidity in adult life.

Betty B. Osman, Ph.D., reviews the co-occurrence of learning disabilities and mental health problems in children and adolescents. The rate of learning disabilities in children referred to mental health centers for behavior problems in school is much higher, about 30%, than is found in the general population. Dr. Osman carefully details the definition of learning disability and its use by the Individuals With Disabilities Education Act (IDEA), the federal law (1990) that reauthorized and encompassed the Education for All Handicapped Children Act (1975). She carefully explores the strengths and weakness of the discrepancy formula and illustrates how the formula can vary from state to state. She then reviews the various theories pertaining to the etiology of learning disabilities, followed by a discussion of the decision to list the learning disabilities under Axis I in DSM-IV (American Psychiatric Association 1994). She explores the epidemiology of learning disability, showing that boys have higher rates of learning disability than do girls. Dr. Osman also introduces the subject of nonverbal learning disabilities and how they worsen over time. She details the effect of learning disabilities on the social-emotional development and how learning disabilities play a role in intensifying the symptoms of a wide variety of child and adolescent psychiatric disorders.

Sally E. Shaywitz, M.D., and her colleagues focus on the cognitive and neurobiological advances in dyslexia and their clinical implications for children and, particularly, young adults with this common disorder. Dr. Shaywitz masterfully reviews the epidemiology, cognitive basis, and neural basis for dyslexia. She then uses state-of-the-art technology to explain how functional magnetic resonance imaging (fMRI) accurately locates the brain areas that show changes in metabolic activity during reading tasks. This noninvasive technique uses no ionizing radiation. This safety factor allows fMRI to be used repeatedly during a reading task. Dr. Shaywitz was able to discern differences between men and women in brain activation during phonological processing. Error patterns on the fMRI tasks revealed that dyslexic persons differed from nonimpaired adult readers most on the nonword rhyme task in key anatomical areas of the postcortical system, including Wernicke's area, the angular gyrus, the extrastriate cortex, and the striate cortex. This provides a neuroanatomical locus unique to phonological processing. Dyslexic readers failed to show systematic modulation in brain activation patterns at that anatomical locus seen in nondyslexic readers. In addition, the fMRI revealed hemispheric differences during reading tasks. Dr. Shaywitz concludes that the brain activation patterns in dyslexic adults provide evidence of an imperfectly functioning system for segmenting words into their phonological constituents. Finally, Dr. Shaywitz provides translational applications of these fMRI findings to help clinicians use educational history as the most sensitive and most accurate indicator of dyslexia. In treating adolescents and young adults in college who have dyslexia, Dr. Shaywitz illustrates how the principle of accommodation (provide extra time on examinations, allow the use of tape recorders) works better than remediation.

James M. Swanson, Ph.D., and colleagues address the shortcomings of the discrepancy definition of learning disabilities. They show how different definitions of learning disability—specifically, contrasting those definitions that include an IQ–achievement test discrepancy with those that do not—select different types of students. If the discrepancy model is used, it biases toward those with higher IQs. If pure achievement score on achievement tests of reading is used, then a much wider range of students is included, specifically, minorities and those whose families have less prestigious occupations. Dr. Swanson and his co-authors use data from the National Institute of Mental Health Multimodal Treatment Study for Attention-Deficit/Hyperactivity Disorder (MTA Study) of 579 children.

Rosemary Tannock, Ph.D., begins her chapter with the observation that problems in various neurodevelopmental domains, such as speech, language, motor skills, and academic functioning (those skills that are disrupted in learning disabilities), in addition to the core behavioral symptoms of inattention and/or hyperactivity-impulsivity, often occur together. The frequent co-occurrence of deficits in attention, motor control, and perception have led to a commonly recognized pattern termed *DAMP*. Related to these are a series of disabilities that disrupt language function, often found in children with attention-deficit/hyperactivity disorder (ADHD)—pragmatic deficits, including excessive verbal output and timing problems in terms of initiating conversation, taking turns, and maintaining or changing topics during conversation. Picking up a topic in Dr. Shaywitz's chapter, Dr. Tannock describes that children with reading disability have core deficits in the oral language skills of phonemic awareness (which refers to the ability to recognize and manipulate the phonemic constituents of speech), naming speed, and motor coordination. These deficits have variable responses to the effects of psychostimulants. Dr. Tannock concludes that stimulant medication has no systematic or robust effects on the type of language, reading, or motor skill problems that accompany ADHD. Dr. Tannock then reviews the evidence for the involvement of the cerebellum in various learning disabilities associated with ADHD. She concludes by stating the importance of including an evaluation of language, reading, and motor skills and inattention/hyperactivity routinely in the assessment of children referred to specialty clinics with this constellation of symptoms. She cautions that these language issues complicate the known effective treatments—stimulants and behavior modification.

In these five chapters, the authors present clear and incontrovertible evidence that learning disabilities create significant impairments in occupational success, educational attainment, and peer relationships that extend across the age span. Early identification and intervention are essential to prevent long-term failure and demoralization.

References

American Psychiatric Association: Diagnostic and Statistical Manual of Mental Disorders, 4th Edition. Washington, DC, American Psychiatric Association, 1994

Lyon GR: Learning Disabilities, The Future of Child Special Education for Students With Disabilities, Vol 6, No 1, Spring 1996, pp 54–76

Suggested Readings

Denckla MB, LeMay M, Chapman CA: Few CT scan abnormalities found even in neurologically impaired learning disabled children. J Learn Disabil 18:132–135, 1985

Fletcher JM, Francis DJ, Shaywitz SE, et al: Intelligent testing and the discrepancy model for children with learning disabilities. Learning Disabilities: Research & Practice 13:186–203, 1998

Lerner JW: Educational interventions in learning disabilities. J Am Acad Child Adolesc Psychiatry 28:326–331, 1989

Lyon GR, Alexander D, Yaffe S: Progress and promise in research in learning disabilities. Learning Disabilities 8:1–6, 1997

Lyon GT, Chhabra V: The current state of science and the future of specific reading disability. Mental Retardation and Developmental Disabilities Research Reviews 2:2–9, 1996

Chapter 1

Children With Uncomplicated Reading Disorders Grown Up

A Prospective Follow-Up Into Adulthood

Rachel G. Klein, Ph.D.
Salvatore Mannuzza, Ph.D.

Learning disorders, as defined in DSM-IV (American Psychiatric Association 1994), include deficits in the development of academic skills, specifically, reading and arithmetic. Both require achievement below that expected for age and intelligence on standardized individual tests, as well as functional impairment associated with these performance decrements. Reading disorders are the most common learning disorders, and it is self-evident that they incur highly significant functional liability because reading skills are a ubiquitous requirement for successful performance in school and other settings.

DSM-IV reports that the estimated prevalence of reading disorder is 4% in U.S. school-age children, but rates vary in population studies. Thus, epidemiological studies report rates from 4% to 9% (Lewis et al. 1994; Malmgren et al. 1999; Rutter et al. 1970; Silva et al. 1985), depending on the definition applied and the geographic area, with lower rates in rural settings. Yet, as many as 15% of a New Zealand birth cohort of 8-year-olds were classified as having reading disabilities based on a common definition of reading dis-

The study was supported, in part, by USPH Grant MH18579 and by Mental Health Clinical Research Center Grant MH30908. The authors gratefully acknowledge the contribution of Suzanne Vosburg who conducted the data analyses.

ability (i.e., reading performance in excess of one standard deviation below the level expected from performance IQ) (Fergusson and Lynskey 1997). These inconsistencies are puzzling, but there is no instance of extremely low frequencies of reading disorder, and it is generally agreed that reading disorders are not rare.

A large literature attests to the relative stability of reading disorders *through childhood* (e.g., Maughan et al. 1985, and reviewed in Beitchman and Young 1997). As with any prevalent and chronic disorder, the long-term costs are a public health concern. These include the effect of reading disorders on educational and occupational attainment, social function, and future psychiatric problems. Understandably, knowledge about the longitudinal course of learning disorders has been deemed a high priority (Raskind et al. 1998).

No controversy exists over the seriousness of dysfunctions associated with reading deficits, and society's concern is well documented through the numerous remedial educational resources that have been developed to address them both in and out of academic centers. However, there has been controversy concerning the effect of reading disorders on the emotional and behavioral adjustment of affected children. The fact that reading disorders are relatively stable through childhood (Maughan et al. 1985) makes it all the more credible that they are likely to have negative consequences on various aspects of children's adjustment through multiple pathways, such as hampering the acquisition of cognitive skills, or through constraints placed on life opportunities because of limited reading skills (Maughan et al. 1985; Stanovich 1994).

Interest in the relation between learning disorders and psychiatric problems has a long history, originally prompted by the observed relation between childhood reading disorders and aggressive behavior (i.e., Berger et al. 1975; Rutter et al. 1970). A common view has held that learning disorders, especially reading disorders, place children at risk for the development of conduct disorder. The co-occurrence of poor academic skills and conduct problems has fostered several explanatory developmental theories (Rutter et al. 1970).

One theory is that behavior problems, with their concomitant interference with school performance, may lead to reading deficits

(DeBaryshe et al. 1993). Another influential hypothesis is that children with learning disorders are at high risk for conduct problems because of their negative school experience. In the face of repeated academic failure, children develop low self-esteem and disengage from a school milieu that brings them only defeat and disappointment. As a result of their disaffection toward the mainstream culture of school, they turn to negative behaviors as a substitute for school-related activities. The pattern represents a concrete example of the proverb that the devil makes work for idle hands. Peer relationships with troubled young people who also devalue school are sought out, setting a cycle of social experience that fosters conduct problems and eventually conduct disorders. Alternatively, neurobiological factors that may influence the development of learning disorders may be related to other childhood disorders. Therefore, biological factors might represent a liability for both learning and conduct disorders. However, if so, risks associated with learning disorders probably would not be limited to antisocial disorders; instead, they would likely be manifest through a variety of psychiatric disorders. In keeping with this model, children with other disorders, such as attention-deficit hyperactivity disorder (ADHD), have been reported to have elevated rates of learning disorders (Semrud-Clikeman et al. 1992).

Because of the noted coexistence of poor school performance and aggression, much of the longitudinal research on the behavioral outcome of children with reading disorders has focused on conduct disorder and delinquency. Relatively elevated rates of delinquency in adolescents with childhood reading disabilities have been reported; however, these were accounted for by socioeconomic and other demographic factors (Keilitz and Dunivant 1986; Wadsworth 1979, in Williams and McGee 1994). In New Zealand, Williams and McGee (1994) found that among boys, reading disability at age 9 years had a modest but significant influence on conduct disorder at age 15 years, even after controlling for other potential influences, including behavioral status at age 9. A strength of this study was the inclusion of psychiatric evaluations and the application of DSM-III (American Psychiatric Association 1980) standards for assessing conduct disorder at ages 9 and 15. Despite the relatively elevated rate of DSM-III diagnoses of conduct disorder, the boys who had reading disorders at age 9 did not have more subsequent police contacts. In addition, their reading disability at age 9 was not related to *ratings* of antisocial behavior completed by their parents and by the adolescents about themselves. Thus, early reading disability was predictive of the diagnosis of conduct disorder but not of other measures of behavioral conflicts in adolescent boys. The results are even more striking because other studies of antisocial behavior have examined rates of delinquency, such as police involvement, or behavioral ratings but have not relied on clinical psychiatric diagnoses as outcome measures.

In contrast to the New Zealand study, another epidemiological study found that childhood reading disability posed a risk for conduct problems, as rated by teachers, but only in girls (Maughan et al. 1996). The results of both studies have been called into question (Fergusson and Lynskey 1997) for failure to take into consideration confounding factors that, when controlled for, remove a straightforward relation between early reading disorders and later conduct problems. These authors correctly noted that inconsistent patterns of results, such as different pathways in girls and boys, can be expected when confounding variables are not taken into consideration.

Despite the emphasis placed on the deleterious consequences of reading disability, few studies of long-term adjustment other than antisocial behavior have been conducted. For example, low "academic" self-esteem, trait anxiety, and depression have been reported as concurrent features of reading disorders in adolescents (Huntington and Bender 1993). However, because these observations do not derive from systematic diagnostic evaluations, their clinical significance is unclear. At the same time, self-ratings of low academic self-esteem and anxiety may reflect a realistic appreciation of the limitations experienced by academically compromised adolescents.

Longitudinal studies that track function over time are key to an understanding of the influence of learning disorders on later function. However, as noted in literature reviews (Cornwall and Bawden 1992; Levine and Nourse 1998), most follow-up studies extend their assessment into childhood or adolescence, and very little information has been reported on the functional status of adults who had reading disorders as children. Also, several follow-up studies have focused on learning disabled high school students. These older groups consist of chronic, stable forms of learning disorders since those who improved sufficiently so that they no longer qualified for the disorder were excluded; consequently, reports of learning disabled adolescents are not directly relevant to an understanding of the course of children identified in childhood. Indeed, they may paint an unduly dark picture of adult outcome.

Another diagnostic limitation is that several longitudinal studies have selected children in special educational settings as a definitional proxy for learning disorders. This approach samples a heterogeneous population of academically compromised children whose dysfunctions are unknown. The inferences that can be drawn from studies of children in special education are complicated further by secular changes in educational policy that have led to changes in the population of children served by special educational resources. Thus, a major interpretive handicap is the lack of systematic diagnostic information at the time learning disorder was diagnosed.

Although most long-term studies have methodological limitations (see Cornwall and Bawden 1992; Maughan 1995), several well-designed longitudinal studies of the behavioral adjustment of children with reading disorders have been done. Unfortunately, they either span a very brief follow-up interval or do not extend into adulthood (McGee et al. 1986, 1988; Sanson et al. 1996; Smart et al. 1996; Spreen 1981). Only a few relevant studies have been reported on the adult adjustment of children with reading disabilities.

To assess the independent and combined influence of reading disorder and conduct problems on school history, as well as on educational attainment and occupational status, a British study examined four groups of carefully identified white 10-year-olds in an inner London population: children with and without well-defined reading disorders and children with and without conduct problems (Maughan et al. 1985). One year after they left school, at ages 17–19 years, those with early childhood reading disorders (regardless of conduct status at age 10 years) were more likely to be unemployed and, if working, to have unskilled jobs. Those with *both* reading and conduct problems in childhood fared significantly worse in both aspects of employment. Those with conduct problems showed the worst outcome after leaving school, but those with prior retarded reading skills were still worse than control subjects. The results highlight the liability imposed on children with early reading disorder, even when conduct problems are not present. Quality of adjustment and psychiatric status at follow-up were not a focus of study.

Another study, drawing from the same population as the above study, examined adjustment in adults (at mean age of nearly 28 years) who had reading disorders at age 10 and in control subjects (Maughan et al. 1996). Adults were assessed for a history of antisocial behavior and criminality, alcoholism, and personality disorders (antisocial or withdrawn). Reading disorders were not associated with elevated rates of any of these dysfunctions. However, despite sampling from a large pool of children, and a remarkably high retrieval rate of 81% 17 years later, few persons had reading disorders in childhood. Because rates of antisocial outcomes were very low in girls, comparisons were restricted to boys: 48 in the reading disorder group and 29 in the control group. Therefore, it is difficult to rule out type II errors in concluding that reading disorders are not associated with later antisocial behavior or alcoholism. However, any relationship is likely to be weak, based on this study's findings.

As noted, limited attention has been given to risks for multiple aspects of clinically assessed psychiatric disorders. A 13-year follow-up Canadian study is the only one to have examined multiple clinical aspects of early adult adjustment in children with specific reading disabilities (Bruck 1985). Of all the children with at least average IQs who were 5 to 10 years old and who had no primary behavior problems when referred to a specialized clinic, 101 were evaluated between ages 17 and 29 (mean age 21 years). Comparison subjects were recruited through the acquaintanceship method, by requesting nominations from participants for relatives and friends of similar ages and social circumstances with no learning disorders. Many control subjects had attained exceptional accomplishments. Therefore, to provide a closer match to the reading disabled individuals, their siblings who had no learning disability in childhood were added to the study. A clinical interview was conducted with the individuals who had reading disabilities, the control subjects, and a parent, but siblings were not clinically assessed. Based on detailed clinical narratives of the interviews, an overall rating of well-being was formulated.

At follow-up, compared with control subjects, those with childhood reading disability had worse reading performance and had received less schooling. Employment status could not be compared because a large proportion of the control subjects were students, but among those employed, occupational status was worse in the disabled group. In contrast, the educational and occupational attainment of the siblings was not better than that of their disabled brothers and sisters. With regard to clinical aspects of adjustment, the reading disabled group was significantly worse than the control subjects, but at follow-up, the individuals with a childhood history of reading problems were not severely impaired, and fewer than 5% were judged to have serious psychiatric disturbance—in general, these young adults were managing well, and even though their peers were better, the two groups did not specifically differ in rates of conduct problems.

Contrary to other findings (Williams and McGee 1994), the girls were reported to have worse outcomes than the boys; however, conclusions about sex differences in adjustment at follow-up are not justified because appropriate analyses were not performed. Unfortunately, the study did not include a definition of reading disability. Also problematic is the comment that 85% of the group with reading disabilities had adjustment problems in childhood, the nature of which was not specified.

The study found, in effect, that the adjustment of most children with reading disabilities improves over time if they had problems in childhood. However, these early problems make it difficult to interpret what accounted for a worse outcome in the clinic children: reading disability or problem behaviors? Other methodological issues include the fact that fewer than 60% of the original group were followed up, that clinical interviews were not conducted blindly (i.e., without knowledge of childhood status), that

IQ measures were not obtained in control subjects or siblings, and that a considerable proportion were still of school age at reevaluation, so that information about adult outcome is incomplete.

Yet, the study (Bruck 1985) has drawn serious attention, and its failure to obtain elevated rates of maladjustment in the young adulthood of children with reading disorders has been influential. The study's importance has stemmed from its comprehensive, systematic assessment of educational and occupational attainment and its ascertainment of clinical status from multiple sources.

In contrast to the findings from the above Canadian study, a large systematic 7-year prospective study of a whole first-grade population in Chicago, Illinois, found that teacher ratings of learning disorders, defined as the teacher's judgment that the child was not learning up to capacity in first grade, predicted relatively higher levels of self-rated depression, anxiety, and overall distress in the teenage boys. Learning disorders in first grade did not predict these outcomes in the girls (Kellam et al. 1983).

As far as we know, no other prospective follow-up studies of clinical outcomes have been done in children with reading disorders. To investigate the course of childhood reading disorders into adulthood, we undertook a prospective longitudinal study of the educational, occupational, and psychiatric status of elementary school–age children with reading disorders but no other psychiatric disorder.

Study Background

In the 1970s, we were interested in testing the then-popular view that the attention-enhancing and "quieting" effects of stimulant medications were specific to children with ADHD (i.e., the notion that these compounds had a paradoxical effect on hyperactive children). The ideal design for a test of this hypothesis would have been to study the effects of psychostimulants in nonhyperactive children. However, this strategy was deemed ethically unsound. One research team was able to conduct such a study by limiting stimulant administration (dextroamphetamine) to a single dose (Rapoport et al. 1978). Although informative, the study of acute doses may not illuminate outcomes associated with chronic drug exposure. To study the response to sustained stimulant treatment in nonhyperactive school-age children, in whom stimulant medication was a reasonable therapeutic intervention, we selected children with learning disorders who showed no evidence of hyperactivity or any other significant psychiatric symptomatology. Stimulant treatment in this population was justifiable because, should the paradoxical effect model be erroneous, the children's attentional capacity might be enhanced, and academic performance might in turn be improved.

Two randomized, placebo-controlled trials of methylphenidate were conducted in children with what we refer to as *uncomplicated reading disorders* (Gittelman et al. 1983; Gittelman-Klein and Klein 1976). The study children with reading disorders constituted the sample followed up into adulthood. Concurrently with the follow-up study of children with reading disorder, our research group was examining the longitudinal course into adulthood of similarly aged children with ADHD, as well as children with separation anxiety disorder, who had been referred by schools to the same clinic. The a priori design was to use the comparison individuals recruited for these parallel follow-up studies as the control subjects for the present longitudinal study of reading disorders.

The clinic where children were referred was located in an outer borough of greater New York with mostly Caucasian residents. Few children from other ethnic groups were referred, so non-Caucasian children were too scarce to represent a meaningful follow-up sample. The same restriction applies to the present investigation of uncomplicated reading disorder.

Study Goals

The study was designed to test the hypothesis that as adults, children with uncomplicated learning disorders, relative to comparisons, would have a significant excess of psychiatric disorder. In addition, the follow-up study included a comprehensive functional assessment that encompassed educational and occupational status to describe outcome in these related functional domains. Some studies have reported contrasting developmental trajectories in boys and girls, with inconsistency in the nature of the sex differences. Although the issue is important, we do not examine sex differences because the number of girls among the children with reading disorder has been deemed too small ($n = 27$) to generate meaningful results.

Methods

Subjects

All subjects—those with uncomplicated reading disorders and control subjects—resided in the same geographic area. Because procedures for identifying male and female control subjects diverged, they are described separately.

Uncomplicated Reading Disorders

The selection process was aimed at the identification of nonretarded children with no psychopathology but with documented reading disorders that interfered with school performance. Reading disorder was defined with a discrepancy method that required decrements between intellectual (IQ) and reading ability. Between 1970 and 1978, the Child Development Clinic of Long Island Jewish Medical Center solicited referrals of children, ages 7 through 12 years, whose teachers judged them as having significant academic but no behavior problems. More than 450 children were screened, of whom 111 Caucasian children (82 boys, 29 girls) met the following criteria:

1. Were referred by their primary school teacher because of academic problems
2. Described through telephone contact with the teacher as presenting no behavior problems in school
3. Rated as not hyperactive by the teacher, defined as a score of less than 1.5 on the Hyperactivity Factor of the Conners Teacher Rating Scale (Conners 1969)
4. Had a Verbal or Performance Wechsler Intelligence Scale for Children—Revised (WISC-R; Wechsler 1974) IQ of at least 85 and a Full-Scale IQ of at least 80 (the Full-Scale IQ requirement was aimed at excluding children who had a very low Verbal or Performance IQ, possibly in the retarded range)

5. Had a reading lag relative to IQ (described later in this chapter)
6. Had no significant psychiatric problems as assessed through a psychiatric evaluation
7. Attended a regular class (children in special education classes were not considered because, at the time, these pupils typically had complex multifaceted difficulties)
8. Had a history of adequate exposure to academic instruction to rule out the possibility that reading problems were, even if only in part, the result of limited environmental opportunity for skill acquisition
9. Had no sensory impairment
10. Had no chronic serious medical illness or neurological disorder
11. Spoke English at home
12. Had a telephone in the home

The latter requirement has been standard in our treatment studies because ready access and communication between the clinic staff and the family is necessary.

As stated earlier in this chapter, the children were evaluated for one of two treatment studies of reading disorders: 1) a placebo-controlled study of methylphenidate (Gittelman-Klein and Klein 1976) and 2) a study of the effects of methylphenidate and reading remediation (Gittelman and Feingold 1983; Gittelman et al. 1983). Both studies required a significant lag in reading, but criteria for this lag differed. The first study required 2 years below grade level on either the Wide Range Achievement Test (WRAT; Jastak and Jastak 1968) or the Gray Oral Reading Test (Gray 1963). The second study required reading below grade level on the WRAT and the Gray Oral Reading Test, depending on IQ, as follows: 1) if Verbal IQ was 85–90, 2.0 years or more; 2) if Verbal IQ was 91–95, 1.5 years or more; 3) if Verbal IQ was 96 or greater, 1.0 year or more.

A clinical social worker obtained detailed histories of the children and of family function. A report of findings and the forms completed by the social worker, parent, and teacher were given to the child psychiatrist before a clinical examination with the child and parent. The psychiatric evaluation was standardized to elicit specific information about motor activity, conduct problems, affect, mood, anxiety, psychotic symptoms, and developmental history. The psychiatrist completed a Children's Psychiatric Rating Scale (National Institute of Mental Health 1973). Only children without clinical disorders, except for specific developmental disorders, were considered for study. In addition, children received a medical examination that included a medical history and a standardized clinical neurological examination.

At the time the children with uncomplicated reading disorders were identified, they were age 10.2 years, on average, and had a mean Full-Scale IQ of 96 (Verbal IQ 96; Performance IQ 97). Their average socioeconomic status (SES) score (range of 1 through 5) (Hollingshead and Redlich 1958) was 3.0 ± 0.9, indicating that, on average, children came from middle- to lower-middle-class backgrounds. Behavioral ratings during childhood on parent and teacher rating scales have been reported (Gittelman and Feingold 1983; Gittelman et al. 1983; Gittelman-Klein and Klein 1976). They indicate very low levels of hyperactivity, conduct problems, or anxiety (i.e., mean scores below 1.0 on factors with score ranges of 0–3). The teacher ratings documented that troublesome behavior was absent at the time their pupils were given a diagnosis of uncomplicated reading disorder.

Male Control Subjects

Male control subjects were identified for a prospective follow-up of children with ADHD, which was conducted concurrently with the current study of children with uncomplicated reading disorders (Gittelman et al. 1985). Because the follow-up of children with ADHD included mostly boys, only male control subjects were identified. The ADHD follow-up study included two waves, the first during the subjects' adolescence and the second in adulthood (Mannuzza et al. 1993). Male control subjects were recruited during the first wave, when they were adolescents. Medical charts from the adolescent medicine outpatient clinic of Long Island Jewish Medical Center were reviewed to identify boys with no recorded behavior problems before age 13 years who were seen at the clinic for routine physical examinations or acute illnesses (e.g., the flu). Individuals treated for accidental injuries or chronic, serious illnesses, or those for whom behavior problems before age

13 were noted in their medical chart, were not pursued. For others, parents were called and asked whether elementary school teachers had ever complained about their child's behavior. If parents reported no teacher complaints before age 13, the boy was recruited if the family fit the SES range that was targeted to correspond to the SES of the children with ADHD. As it happened, the children with ADHD and those with uncomplicated reading disorder had similar SES; therefore, the procedure implemented led to analogous SES in the uncomplicated reading disorder and the male comparison groups.

The 100 male control subjects were white and ages 16–23 years at wave 1 of the follow-up study of the ADHD children (mean ± SD: age, 18.9 ± 1.5; SES, 3.1 ± 1.0).

Female Control Subjects

Female control subjects, who were adults at the time of the study, were recruited for a prospective longitudinal study of children with separation anxiety disorder who had been referred because of school refusal (Gittelman-Klein and Klein 1971, 1973). Control subjects were recruited through random-digit dialing in the areas where schools that had referred children to the clinic were located. Homes were called, the study was explained briefly to the respondent, and the respondent was asked about the presence of a woman within the appropriate age range. When someone in the household met the age criterion, sociodemographic information, such as race and parental SES, was obtained. If a match was made, the respondent was asked if she had ever had school difficulties during elementary school. If not, the person was recruited. A total of 34 female control subjects were enrolled.

Adult Follow-Up Assessment

Letters were sent to potential participants informing them of the study and to anticipate a call. The recruiting social worker explained the study to participants over the telephone and obtained verbal consent. Interviewers obtained written informed consent before the evaluation. Efforts were made to interview all subjects directly; when this was not possible, we interviewed an informant, regularly the mother. Subjects were given a semistructured clinical psychiatric interview that elicited DSM-III-R (American Psychiatric Association 1987) lifetime histories for diagnoses of antisocial personality, attention-deficit, anxiety, mood, substance use, and psychotic disorders (Mannuzza and Klein 1987). Because interviewers were instructed and trained to pursue any clinical leads, some diagnoses were made that were not part of the schedule. Blind assessments were conducted by clinical psychologists and a psychiatric social worker, who received extensive training in differential diagnosis and who achieved good to excellent reliability on major disorders (Mannuzza et al. 1993). The interview schedule also included systematic inquiry about academic, occupational, and social history and functioning. If a subject was not available, efforts were made to obtain an informant interview with a parent. The procedures applied were identical to self and informant clinical interviews.

Interviewers wrote clinical narratives that included general information (e.g., marital status, living circumstances, job history) and that documented all diagnoses, specifying their age at onset and offset and level of diagnostic certainty. Blindly, narratives were checked (by S.M.) for diagnostic accuracy and completeness, and diagnostic dilemmas were reviewed by the authors.

Adult Psychiatric Status

Probable and definite DSM-III-R diagnoses were made. Probable diagnoses consisted of conditions that did not meet the full complement of diagnostic criteria required to qualify for a diagnosis, but symptoms were associated with clear functional impairment or distress. Definite diagnoses met full symptom criteria with impairment. Probable and definite diagnoses are combined in this report because this procedure is consistent with clinical practice in that functional disruption was required regularly for any diagnosis.

The focus of this chapter is on mental disorders. These were classified as current if they had been active up to 2 months prior to the follow-up. The only exceptions were personality and substance use disorders, which were considered ongoing if they had occurred within the antecedent 6 months. For completeness sake, we report on current and previous mental disorders; namely, those that had occurred at any time during the person's life but that were no longer present at follow-up. Having a full picture of the children's psychiatric history is potentially informative because a multiwave longitudinal study of children with reading disorders found that, in contrast to control subjects, they had significantly higher rates of dysfunction at midpoint and in late childhood than in adolescence (McGee et al. 1992).

In addition to eliciting information about symptoms, inquiry extended to general aspects of the person's life, and the clinical interviewers formulated ratings of overall adjustment and effectiveness in school-related activities, in the workplace, and in social and marital relationships. These ratings were completed for adolescence (defined as up to age 18) and for adulthood.

Data Analyses

Student t tests for independent groups were applied to contrasts of continuous measures, and χ^2 was applied to dichotomous variables. Because of IQ differences between the uncomplicated reading disorder and comparison groups reported below in the "Results" section, we examined whether IQ at follow-up was related to the presence of a mental disorder, other than a specific learning disorder. None of the IQs at follow-up (Verbal, Performance, or Full-Scale) was significantly associated with the presence of a diagnosis ($P = 0.41$–0.92). As a result, contrasts for mental disorders were not adjusted for IQ. In contrast, it is well established that intellectual (IQ) and academic skills are not independent. Therefore, the group comparisons for reading and arithmetic test performance controlled for IQ by means of analysis of covariance (ANCOVA). P values reported are all two-tailed probability tests.

Results

Length of Follow-Up and Retrieval Rate

The follow-up interval was 16 years. Information was obtained from 105 of the 111 children with uncomplicated reading disorders (94.6%). Three could not be located (2 males, 1 female),

2 refused (1 male, 1 female), and 1 jailed subject could not be evaluated. One of the males in the uncomplicated reading disorder group was deceased, and an informant interview was obtained. Interview data were lost for 1 male, so we report on 104 of the original 111 cases (93.7%). Of 100 male control subjects recruited in adolescence, 95 (95%) were followed up into adulthood. Because the female control subjects were obtained at the adult follow-up, retrieval rate is not an issue. Informant diagnostic interviews were obtained in 40 of the 104 individuals in the uncomplicated reading disorder group (38.5%) and in 34 of the 129 control subjects (26.4%).

Subject Characteristics at Follow-Up

Table 1–1 shows demographic characteristics at 16-year follow-up.

Table 1–1. Demographic characteristics of reading disorder and comparison groups in adulthood at 16-year follow-up

	Reading disorder (n = 104)		Comparison (n = 129)		t or χ^2	$P*$
Sex	**Male**	**Female**	**Male**	**Female**		
	77 (74%)	27 (26%)	95 (74%)	34 (26%)	0.01	0.95
Age [years; mean (SD)]	26.1 (2.4)		27.0 (2.5)		–2.98	0.003
Age range (years)	20–31		23–34			
Socioeconomic status[a] [mean (SD)]	3.08 (0.84)		2.70 (0.90)		3.29	0.001
Marital status						
Single (never married)	71 (68%)		71 (55%)		4.84	0.09
Married	27 (26%)		51 (40%)			
Divorced or separated	6 (6%)		7 (5%)			

*Two-tailed P values.
[a]Hollingshead and Redlich (1958) two-factor scale.

The group with reading disorders was significantly younger than the comparison group ($P = 0.003$); however, the difference was less than 1 year. No significant group difference in marital status was found, but the reading disorder group tended to have married less often than the comparison group (27% vs. 40%) ($P = 0.09$). Divorce rates were low in both groups (see Table 1–1). At follow-up, at the average age of 26, the uncomplicated reading disorder group had a mean SES level (3.08 ± 0.84) virtually identical to their parents' SES when they were referred by their elementary school teachers. At follow-up, the control subjects' SES (2.70 ± 0.90, $P = 0.001$) was significantly better than the SES of their reading disabled peers. Because the groups originally came from similar socioeconomic levels, the disadvantage at follow-up in the former clinic children reflects that, relative to parental status, the reading disordered subjects had remained stagnant, whereas the male control subjects had moved forward. As expected, IQ was significantly lower in the group with childhood reading disorders ($P = 0.000$). The group's IQ had declined over time since childhood when, as noted above, the group's average WISC-R Full-Scale IQ was 96.

Educational Attainment and Academic Test Performance

As anticipated based on the literature, educational attainment was much worse in the adults with early reading disorders relative to control subjects (see Table 1–2). Even controlling for IQ, the uncomplicated reading disorder subjects had significantly worse performance in reading and arithmetic ($P = 0.000$). Their low attainment indicates clinically significant functional impairment in reading ability. The WRAT reading level of the uncomplicated reading disorder group was 12 points below IQ, whereas this was not the case for the comparison group.

Occupational Status

Employment rates were high in both groups. Although a similar proportion of the uncomplicated reading disorder and comparison groups was employed at follow-up (78% and 88%, respectively), the difference reached statistical significance ($P = 0.05$) (Table 1–3).

Table 1–2. Educational status of reading disorder and comparison groups in adulthood at 16-year follow-up

	Reading disorder (n = 104) N (%)	Comparison (n = 129) N (%)	t, F, or χ^2	P*
Education				
No high school diploma or general equivalency diploma	28 (27)	5 (4)	53.66	0.000
General equivalency diploma	9 (9)	8 (6)		
High school graduate	60 (58)	59 (46)		
College graduate	7 (7)	47 (36)		
Advanced degree	0 (0)	10 (8)		
WAIS-R IQ[a] [mean (SD)]				
Full-Scale IQ	87.2 (8.5)	109.9 (14.9)	−11.70	0.000
Range	73–112	75–137		
Verbal IQ	86.4 (7.7)	110.0 (14.2)	−12.84	0.000
Range	73–106	77–137		
Performance IQ	91.2 (11.5)	108.5 (15.7)	−8.10	0.000
Range	68–121	74–138		
WRAT-R[b] [mean (SD)]				
Reading Standard score	75.2 (14.5)	108.9 (15.5)	53.56	0.000
Range	46–104	64–138		
Arithmetic Standard score	76.8 (14.2)	98.4 (14.4)	4.08	0.05
Range	50–112	67–128		

*Two-tailed P values.
[a]Wechsler Adult Intelligence Scale—Revised (Wechsler 1981).
[b]Wide Range Achievement Test—Revised (Jastak and Jastak 1983). Analyses of covariance were carried out with Full-Scale IQ as the covariate.

Significantly more uncomplicated reading disorder subjects than control subjects were temporarily unemployed at follow-up (about one in nine; $P = 0.02$), but few (4%) were on public assistance.

Although employment rates were similar in the two groups, occupational level was not. As expected, the children with

Table 1–3. Occupational status of reading disorder and comparison groups in adulthood at 16-year follow-up

	Reading disorder (*n* = 104) *N* (%)	Comparison (*n* = 129) *N* (%)	χ^2	*P**
Current job status				
Full-time	77 (74)	101 (78)	0.58	0.45
Part-time	4 (4)	12 (9)	2.68	0.10
Student	3 (3)	5 (4)	0.17	0.68
Housewife	5 (5)	4 (3)	0.45	0.50
Supported by someone (e.g., alimony)	0 (0)	1 (1)	0.81	0.37
Unemployed (temporarily)	11 (11)	4 (3)	5.34	0.02
Unemployed (welfare)	4 (4)	2 (2)	1.21	0.27
Overall χ^2			10.22	0.12
Occupational level[a]				
Higher executive, owner of large or medium concern, major or lesser professional	4 (4)	40 (31)	27.73	0.001
Administrative, owner of small business, minor professional, clerical or sales worker, technician	42 (40)	55 (43)	0.12	0.73
Skilled manual, semiskilled, machine operator	51 (49)	30 (23)	16.88	0.001
Unskilled	5 (5)	4 (3)	0.45	0.50
Not relevant (never employed)	2 (2)	0 (0)	2.50	0.11
Overall χ^2			36.49	0.001

*Two-tailed *P* values.
[a]Hollingshead and Redlich (1958) occupational categories.

Table 1–4. Characteristics of histories of reading disorder and comparison groups in adulthood at 16-year follow-up

	Reading disorder ($n = 104$) N (%)	Comparison ($n = 129$) N (%)	χ^2	P*
Currently employed	81 (78)	113 (88)	3.90	0.05
Job problems since age 18				
Not applicable	3 (3)	0 (0)	6.93	0.07
None	83 (80)	99 (77)		
Occasionally	16 (15)	21 (16)		
Frequently	2 (2)	9 (7)		
Quit a job since age 18				
Not applicable	3 (3)	0 (0)	4.48	0.21
Never	71 (68)	97 (75)		
Once	22 (21)	24 (19)		
At least twice	8 (8)	8 (6)		
Fired since age 18				
Not applicable	3 (3)	0 (0)	5.62	0.13
Never	84 (81)	102 (79)		
Once	15 (14)	20 (16)		
At least twice	2 (2)	7 (5)		

*Two-tailed P values.

uncomplicated reading disorder, as adults, held lower-level positions ($P = 0.001$) and were more often in semiskilled jobs, relative to the comparison group ($P = 0.001$).

As evident from Table 1–4, despite clear disadvantage in occupational attainment, the children with reading disorders were not significantly worse than control subjects with regard to job problems or being fired.

Psychiatric Status at Follow-Up

Table 1–5 presents the rate of current mental disorders at follow-up. The poor readers had significantly more mood and substance

Table 1–5. Current diagnoses[a] in reading disorder and comparison groups at 16-year follow-up

	Reading disorder (n = 104) N (%)	Comparison (n = 129) N (%)	χ^2	P*
Antisocial personality disorder	4 (4)	2 (2)	1.21	0.27
Mood disorders[b]	6 (6)	1 (1)	4.93	0.03
Substance use disorders	21 (20)	12 (9)	5.62	0.02
Alcohol	17 (16)	10 (8)	4.15	0.04
Drug[c]	9 (9)	4 (3)	3.37	0.07
Anxiety disorders[d]	5 (5)	3 (2)	1.07	0.30
Attention-deficit/ hyperactivity disorder	0 (0)	0 (0)	—	—
Developmental disorders	13 (13)	1 (1)	14.02	0.000
Reading	11 (11)	1 (1)	11.32	0.001
Arithmetic	4 (4)	0 (0)	5.05	0.03
Schizotypal personality disorder	1 (1)	0 (0)	1.25	0.26
Any diagnosis	34 (33)	18 (14)	11.66	0.001
Any diagnosis other than developmental disorders	27 (26)	17 (13)	6.14	0.01

*Two-tailed P values.
[a]Probable and definite DSM-III-R diagnoses.
[b]Mood disorders at follow-up include major depression, dysthymia, and bipolar disorder, not otherwise specified.
[c]Drug use disorders other than alcohol-related disorders.
[d]Anxiety disorders at follow-up include panic disorder, social phobia, simple phobia, obsessive-compulsive disorder, and anxiety disorder not otherwise specified.

use disorders ($P = 0.02$). There was only a trend for drug use disorders (other than alcohol) to be higher in the uncomplicated reading disorder group (9% vs. 3%, $P = 0.07$), but rates of alcohol-related disorders were significantly more prevalent in the former clinic children (16% vs. 8%, $P = 0.04$). In addition, specific developmental disorders were significantly more frequent at follow-up

Table 1–6. Previous diagnoses[a] excluding current disorders among reading disorder and comparison groups at 16-year follow-up

	Reading disorder (n = 104) N (%)	Comparison (n = 129) N (%)	χ^2	P*
Antisocial personality disorder	0 (0)	2 (2)	1.63	0.20
Mood disorders[b]	9 (9)	32 (25)	10.36	0.001
Substance use disorders	30 (29)	44 (34)	0.74	0.39
Alcohol	15 (14)	25 (19)	1.00	0.32
Drug[c]	25 (24)	31 (24)	0.00	1.00
Anxiety disorders[d]	8 (8)	8 (6)	0.20	0.66
Attention-deficit/ hyperactivity disorder	0 (0)	0 (0)	—	—
Any diagnosis other than developmental disorders	41 (39)	63 (49)	2.07	0.15

*Two-tailed P values.
[a]Lifetime probable and definite DSM-III-R diagnoses that were no longer current at follow-up.
[b]Mood disorders at follow-up included major depression and dysthymia.
[c]Drug use disorders other than alcohol-related disorders.
[d]Anxiety disorders before the follow-up include social phobia, separation anxiety disorder, and posttraumatic stress disorder.

among the reading disorder subjects (13% vs. 1%), but the absolute rate was not high.

Table 1–6 presents the relative frequencies of disorders that were not current (i.e., had not been present in the past 2 months) but that had previously occurred. A different picture emerges when these data are compared with current status. Mood disorders were significantly more frequent among the comparison group than the uncomplicated reading disorder group (25% vs. 9%, P = 0.001). No other diagnosis differed between the two groups. By definition, all adults in the uncomplicated reading disorder group had a prior reading disorder, and 13% were so diagnosed at follow-up compared with 1% of the control subjects. In contrast, no single individual in the comparison group was considered to have had a prior reading disorder.

Global Clinician Ratings of Academic, Occupational, and Social Functioning

Global ratings of academic, occupational, and social functioning, made by the clinician on the basis of all information obtained, are shown in Table 1–7. The blind ratings of adjustment in adolescence and adulthood show significant deficits across the board in the uncomplicated reading disorder individuals (all $P = 0.000$).

Table 1–7. Mean global clinical ratings of academic, occupational, and social functioning in reading disorder and comparison groups

	Reading disorder ($n = 104$)	Comparison ($n = 129$)	t	P*
Adolescence				
Academic	4.56 (1.09)	3.27 (1.37)	7.74	0.000
Occupational	4.28 (0.52)	3.31 (0.86)	9.82	0.000
Social	4.15 (0.65)	3.43 (0.98)	6.46	0.000
Adulthood				
Occupational	4.23 (0.61)	3.16 (1.06)	9.02	0.000
Social	4.11 (0.68)	3.40 (0.98)	6.18	0.000

Note. Ratings: 1 = superior, 2 = very good, 3 = good, 4 = average, 5 = fair, 6 = poor. Standard deviations appear in parentheses.
*Two-tailed P values.

Discussion

The study examined the adult psychiatric status of children with reading disorders who did not show significant psychiatric disorders of any type, referred to as uncomplicated reading disorder. The children were judged free of conduct problems, including hyperactivity, based on parent and teacher rating scales. The study had the unique feature of conducting psychiatric examinations to confirm the absence of any mental disorder in the children with a specific reading disorder diagnosis. Evaluations at the 16-year follow-up were conducted without knowledge of childhood history. Moreover, the retrieval rate of almost 95% was high, so that results are not distorted by missing subjects whose outcome is unknown and may differ from that of the participants.

Limitations of longitudinal studies have been reviewed extensively, most recently by Maughan (1995). These include imprecise characterizations of subjects and of definitions of reading disorders, lack of appropriate comparisons, and high attrition rates.

The present study had well-characterized subjects with regard to their early behavioral status, IQ, and reading attainment; however, the control subjects, although evaluated at the same time as the subjects with reading disorders, were derived for other investigative purposes, were not recruited at the same time as the children with reading delays, and were not screened to be exact matches to the clinic patients. However, as children, the subjects with reading disorders and control subjects attended the same neighborhood schools and had equivalent family SES. Nevertheless, the question arises whether standards for enrolling the control subjects could have affected the group contrasts systematically. The control subjects were recruited if they had no evidence of school-related behavior problems, but no attempt was made to exclude those who had reading disorders. To the extent that these occurred, they would have worked against finding a worse outcome for the group with reading disorders. It seems unlikely that this situation occurred because this study's results with regard to academic, occupational, and social outcomes are completely consistent with previous reports. Among the individuals who had reading disorders in childhood, we found disadvantaged educational and occupational attainment, as others have reported. The unique aspect of this study, the determination of psychiatric status of children with well-established pure reading disorders, is not likely to have been compromised because findings from other domains are valid.

The study was not designed to address several issues pertinent to the course of reading disorders. For example, we did not examine the cognitive impairments associated with adult status or the exact nature of the reading disorders in adulthood (although we did so at the time of initial assessment). From a methodological viewpoint, the study's follow-up evaluations were designed to protect the blind and therefore had to match what was being done in the concurrent longitudinal study of children with ADHD. At the same time, the major goal of determining psychiatric history was well served because the focus of the evaluations was on a comprehensive clinical assessment to determine the risks for mental disorders in children whose reading disorders had functional consequences significant enough to warrant teacher referrals. This process is time-consuming for school personnel and is not implemented typically for trivial or transient academic problems.

At follow-up, 16 years after the reading disorders were identified, more than 25% of the children had failed to obtain the minimal academic accomplishment of a high school diploma. In comparison, only 4% of the control subjects had this negative outcome. Fewer than 10% of the children with reading problems obtained a bachelor's degree, and none went on to graduate education. These educational limitations are understandable given the unsatisfactory reading ability of the clinic group. An average standardized reading score of 75 on an untimed word recognition test (WRAT) represents a major handicap for successful educational progress. In view of these poor reading scores, one wonders why more of the reading disorders did not meet DSM-III-R criteria in the adults. There is no clear answer, but it seems likely that the early reading problems posed obstacles to intellectual development so that the adults' IQs were relatively low: on average, only 87.2. It is likely that, in many reading-impaired individuals, the discrepancy between IQ and reading scores probably fell just short of meeting criteria. The issue of what standards to apply to define reading disability in children has been extensively debated, with many arguing against using discrepancy criteria. Because adult IQ is in part affected by a lifetime of reading, determining the sensible means of defining reading disorders becomes even more complex with age. The criteria for diagnosing reading disorders do not appear to do justice to reading handicaps in adults.

The employment history of the children with reading disorders is more optimistic. Although significantly fewer were employed, the difference in employment rate was relatively trivial—only 10% ($P = 0.05$). Also, although more were temporarily unemployed at follow-up, the absolute rate was not strikingly elevated—only 11% as compared with 3% among the control subjects ($P = 0.02$). Temporary unemployment seems more probable in occupations requiring low-level skills. Because the adults with reading disorder were overrepresented in this type of employment, they probably were more likely to have job instability than were the control subjects in higher-level employment. On the whole, however, reading disorders did not lead to failure to be gainfully employed, although less remunerative jobs ensued. As a result, the reading-disabled group failed to follow the generational upward drift in SES characteristic of the U.S. population at the time of the study, especially in the New York area.

Our findings on adjustment are consistent with the expectation that there is a toll exacted in multiple areas of life for children who start out with reading problems. They not only have less academic and occupational success, as can be anticipated, but their social relationships are also less satisfactory as judged by clinicians. The mechanisms that may be responsible for this disadvantage are not clear. They may be related to lower self-esteem, which we did not assess systematically and which is difficult to quantify satisfactorily.

This study's findings are consistent with those reported by Bruck (1985) in her 13-year follow-up, but the early behavioral status of the sample with reading disorders is unclear, except for the absence of primary behavior disorders. In the present study, we found no evidence that pure reading disorders portend antisocial outcomes. In adulthood, current antisocial disorder in the reading disorder group was infrequent (4%) and no different from that in control subjects (2%) or what would be expected in the general population. However, mood disorders were more frequent at follow-up among the clinic patients (6% vs. 1%, $P = 0.03$, Table 1–5). It is difficult to make sense of this finding because the reverse was true for past mood disorders that were reported to have occurred, but these had desisted by the time of follow-up in 25% of the control subjects as compared with 9% of the reading disorder subjects. These counterintuitive results require replication before they can be interpreted with any confidence. No single case of ADHD was diagnosed in either group at any time; nevertheless, we report on this disorder because the result highlights the success of the study's selection process that aimed to exclude children with ADHD. We obtained very different lifetime rates of

ADHD in our follow-up of adults who had ADHD in childhood (Mannuzza et al. 1993).

Despite the absence of antisocial personality disorders that are regularly linked to substance use disorders, the children with reading disorders had twice the rate of alcohol use than the non-reading group at follow-up (16% vs. 8%, $P = 0.04$, Table 1–5). A similar trend occurred for drugs other than alcohol (9% vs. 3%, $P = 0.07$). In our follow-up of children with ADHD, we found in two independent samples that the maintenance of childhood ADHD into adolescence, coupled with the development of conduct disorders in adolescence, mediated and accounted for the onset of substance use disorders. The developmental trajectory in the reading disorder group was clearly different. It is clear that antisocial disorder is not a necessary condition for developing substance abuse. As far as we know, the present sample is the only one in which an excess of these disorders has been found in children with reading disorders. However, Bruck's (1985) follow-up study, which did not report an excess of drug use or abuse, was in a different geographic area (Canada) at a different time—two factors that influence the prevalence of drug use and abuse. The same considerations apply to the comprehensive British study in London that failed to find elevated rates of alcohol problems among retarded readers at age 28 years compared with nonretarded peers (Maughan et al. 1996). We examined whether alcohol problems in our sample were related to the subjects being more commonly single because single individuals may be more prone to use bars as social vehicles than those in conjugal homes would (this possibility was suggested to us by Lee N. Robins, Ph.D.). We found no relation between marital status and alcohol problems. Kellam and associates' (1983) 7-year follow-up of first graders in inner Chicago, an area in which drug use is to be expected, found no relation between teacher-rated early learning problems and later substance abuse. However, the young people may not have been old enough to provide a full opportunity for examining their ultimate pattern of drug use.

This study does not support the hypothesis that childhood reading disorders presage antisocial adjustment at all. However, we found risks for other psychiatric liability. Their exact nature may vary from sample to sample because group differences, even when significant, do not indicate major excesses of dysfunction in the adults with early reading disorder. In many ways, the adult adjustment of these individuals has been compromised, but whether the pathway to dysfunction is through the educational limitations and chronic academic disadvantage that are the usual concomitants of reading disorders is unclear. If so, it would become all the more critical to implement systematic means of identifying children with reading disorders within schools and to institute remedial programs. These likely would have to stretch into late adolescence, at least for a sizable proportion. Of course, any treatment approach, no matter how well intentioned, requires systematic efficacy testing through randomized controlled trials, with blind independent assessments.

References

American Psychiatric Association: Diagnostic and Statistical Manual of Mental Disorders, 3rd Edition. Washington, DC, American Psychiatric Association, 1980

American Psychiatric Association: Diagnostic and Statistical Manual of Mental Disorders, 3rd Edition, Revised. Washington, DC, American Psychiatric Association, 1987

American Psychiatric Association: Diagnostic and Statistical Manual of Mental Disorders, 4th Edition. Washington, DC, American Psychiatric Association, 1994

Beitchman JH, Young AR: Learning disorders with a special emphasis on reading disorders: a review of the past 10 years. J Am Acad Child Adolesc Psychiatry 36:1020–1032, 1997

Berger M, Yule W, Rutter M: Attainment and adjustment in two geographical areas, II: the prevalence of specific reading retardation. Br J Psychiatry 126:510–519, 1975

Bruck M: The adult functioning of children with specific learning disabilities: a follow-up study, in Advances in Applied Developmental Psychology, Vol 1. Edited by Siegel IE. Norwood, NJ, Ablex, 1985, pp 91–129

Conners CK: A teacher rating scale for use in drug studies with children. Am J Psychiatry 126:884–888, 1969

Cornwall A, Bawden HN: Reading disabilities and aggression: a critical review. J Learn Disabil 25:281–288, 1992

DeBaryshe BD, Patterson GR, Capaldi DM: A performance model for academic achievement in early adolescent boys. Dev Psychol 29:795–804, 1993

Fergusson DM, Lynskey MT: Early reading difficulties and later conduct problems. J Child Psychol Psychiatry 38:899–907, 1997

Gittelman R, Feingold I: Children with reading disorders, I: efficacy of reading remediation. J Child Psychol Psychiatry 24:167–191, 1983

Gittelman R, Klein DF, Feingold I: Children with reading disorders, II: effects of methylphenidate in combination with reading remediation. Arch Gen Psychiatry 24:193–212, 1983

Gittelman R, Mannuzza S, Shenker R, et al: Hyperactive boys almost grown up, I: psychiatric status. Arch Gen Psychiatry 42:937–947, 1985

Gittelman-Klein R, Klein DF: Controlled imipramine treatment of school phobia. Arch Gen Psychiatry 25:204–207, 1971

Gittelman-Klein R, Klein DF: School phobia: diagnostic considerations in the light of imipramine effects. J Nerv Ment Dis 156:199–215, 1973

Gittelman-Klein R, Klein DF: Methylphenidate effects in learning disabilities: psychometric changes. Arch Gen Psychiatry 33:655–664, 1976

Gray WS: Gray Oral Reading Test. Indianapolis, IN, Bobbs Merrill, 1963

Hollingshead AB, Redlich FC: Social Class and Mental Illness: A Community Study. New York, John Wiley & Sons, 1958

Huntington DD, Bender WN: Adolescents with learning disabilities at risk? emotional well-being, depression, suicide. J Learn Disabil 26:159–166, 1993

Jastak JF, Jastak SR: Wide Range Achievement Test (WRAT). Wilmington, DE, Jastak Associates, 1968

Jastak JF, Jastak SR: Wide Range Achievement Test—Revised (WRAT-R). Wilmington, DE, Jastak Associates, 1983

Keilitz I, Dunivant N: The relationship between learning disability and juvenile delinquency: current state of knowledge. Remedial and Special Education 7:18–26, 1986

Kellam SG, Brown CH, Rubin BR, et al: Paths leading to teenage psychiatric symptoms and substance use: developmental epidemiological studies in Woodlawn, in Childhood Psychopathology and Development. Edited by Guze SB, Earls FJ, Barrett JE. New York, Raven, 1983, pp 17–47

Levine P, Nourse SW: What follow-up studies say about postschool life for young men and women with learning disabilities: a critical look at the literature. J LearnDisabil 31:212–233, 1998

Lewis C, Hitch GJ, Walker P: The prevalence of specific arithmetic difficulties and specific reading difficulties in 9- to 10-year old boys and girls. J Child Psychol Psychiatry 35:283–292, 1994

Malmgren K, Abbott RD, Hawkins JD: LD and delinquency: rethinking the "link." J Learn Disabil 32:194–200, 1999

Mannuzza S, Klein RG: Schedule for the Assessment of Conduct, Hyperactivity, Anxiety, Mood, and Psychoactive Substances (CHAMPS). New Hyde Park, NY, Children's Behavior Disorders Clinic, Long Island Jewish Medical Center, 1987

Mannuzza S, Klein RG, Bessler A, et al: Adult outcome of hyperactive boys: educational achievement, occupational rank, and psychiatric status. Arch Gen Psychiatry 50:565–576, 1993

Maughan B: Annotation: long-term outcomes of developmental reading problems. J Child Psychol Psychiatry 36:357–371, 1995

Maughan B, Gray G, Rutter M: Reading retardation and antisocial behaviour: a follow-up into employment. J Child Psychol Psychiatry 26:741–758, 1985

Maughan B, Pickles A, Hagell A, et al: Reading problems and antisocial behaviour: developmental trends in comorbidity. J Child Psychol Psychiatry 37:405–418, 1996

McGee R, Williams S, Share DL, et al: The relationship between specific reading retardation, general reading backwardness, and behavioural problems in a large sample of Dunedin boys: a longitudinal study from five to eleven years. J Child Psychol Psychiatry 27:597–610, 1986

McGee R, Share D, Moffitt TE, et al: Reading disability, behaviour problems and juvenile delinquency, in Individual Differences in Children and Adolescents: International Perspectives. Edited by Saklofske DH, Eysenck SBG. London, England, Hodder & Stoughton, 1988, pp 158–172

McGee R, Feehan M, Williams S, et al: DSM-III disorders from age 11 to age 15 years. J Am Acad Child Adolesc Psychiatry 31:50–59, 1992

National Institute of Mental Health Psychopharmacology Research Branch: ECDEU Assessment Battery for Pediatric Psychiatry: Children's Psychiatric Rating Scale (OMB No 68-RO955). Rockville, MD, U.S. Department of Health, Education, and Welfare, 1973

Rapoport JL, Buchsbaum MS, Zahn TP, et al: Dextroamphetamine: cognitive and behavioral effects in normal prepubertal boys. Science 199:560–563, 1978

Raskind MH, Gerber PJ, Goldberg RJ, et al: Longitudinal research in learning disabilities: report on an international symposium. J Learn Disabil 31:266–277, 1998

Rutter M, Tizard J, Whitmore K: Education, Health and Behaviour. London, England, Longman, 1970

Sanson A, Prior M, Smart D: Reading disabilities with and without behaviour problems at 7–8 years: prediction from longitudinal data from infancy to 6 years. J Child Psychol Psychiatry 37:529–541, 1996

Semrud-Clikeman M, Biederman J, Sprich-Buckminster D, et al: Comorbidity between ADDH and learning disability: a review and report in a clinically referred sample. J Am Acad Child Adolesc Psychiatry 31:439–448, 1992

Silva PA, McGee R, Williams S: Some characteristics of 9-year-old boys with general reading backwardness and specific reading retardation. J Child Psychol Psychiatry 26:407–421, 1985

Smart D, Sanson A, Prior M: Connections between reading disability and behavior problems: testing temporal and causal hypotheses. J Abnorm Psychol 24:363–383, 1996

Spreen O: The relationship between learning disability, neurological impairment, and delinquency: results of a follow-up study. J Nerv Ment Dis 169:791–799, 1981

Stanovich KE: Does dyslexia exist? J Child Psychol Psychiatry 35:579–596, 1994

Wadsworth M: Roots of Delinquency: Infancy, Adolescence and Crime. Oxford, England, Martin Robertson, 1979

Wechsler D: Wechsler Intelligence Scale for Children—Revised (WISC-R). New York, Psychological Corporation, 1974

Wechsler D: Wechsler Adult Intelligence Scale—Revised (WAIS-R). New York, Psychological Corporation, 1981

Williams S, McGee R: Reading attainment and juvenile delinquency. J Child Psychol Psychiatry 35:441–459, 1994

Chapter 2

Learning Disabilities and the Risk of Psychiatric Disorders in Children and Adolescents

Betty B. Osman, Ph.D.

The co-occurrence of learning disabilities and mental health problems has been well documented in the past decade (Boetsch et al. 1996; Fergusson and Lynskey; Prior 1996). Although the two kinds of problems can exist independently, the overlap between them has been estimated at 40%–50%, depending on the specific problems considered and the criteria used for assessment (Cantwell and Baker 1991; Maag and Reid 1994). Although estimates vary, it has been suggested that as many as one-third of children and adolescents referred to mental health centers for behavior problems in school have undiagnosed learning disabilities (Cohen et al. 1993; Kauffman 1997; Little 1993).

Both clinical and epidemiological data suggest that various types of learning disabilities are likely to co-occur (Hallahan and Kauffman 1997) and also that they are frequently comorbid with Axis I psychiatric syndromes (i.e., attention-deficit disorders, adjustment disorders, anxiety, and depression) (Cantwell and Baker 1991). Even when the criteria for an Axis I diagnosis are not met, however, performance anxiety, social skills deficits, low self-esteem, and learned helplessness are likely to co-occur (Kauffman 1997; Kavale and Forness 1995). Furthermore, in children who do have psychiatric disorders, the presence of comorbid learning disabilities predicts the continued presence, rather than the remission, of the psychiatric disorder.

The nature of the relation between emotional and learning disorders has not been emphasized in research. Studies on the development of learning disabilities tend to focus on cognitive and perceptual aspects, whereas research on psychological problems centers on interactional family and social precursors.

Elucidation of the learning-emotional connection is important both for the theoretical understanding of the etiology of learning and behavioral disorders and for the practical development of the most effective educational and clinical interventions.

Yet despite the evidence of co-occurrence, federal regulations and state guidelines discourage comorbid diagnoses. Although the use of multiple diagnoses is not explicitly prohibited, federal reimbursements to state and local agencies are based on the number of students identified, not on the total number of handicapping conditions identified (Rothstein 1990). The original intent of this ruling was fiscal control, but its effect has been a reluctance by states and school districts to acknowledge multiple diagnoses, thereby restricting educational programs.

In this chapter, I review the current understanding of learning disabilities and their status as risk factors for psychiatric disorders.

Learning Disabilities

Learning disabilities are among the most commonly identified developmental problems of childhood today, occurring in approximately 4%–5% of the school-age population in the United States (Beitchman and Young 1997). In spite of this prevalence, and in spite of the federal laws in place to address these disorders in schools, the definitions and the diagnostic criteria used to classify these disabilities continue to be controversial (Beitchman and Young 1997; Kavale and Forness 1995; Prior 1996). This lack of consensus has obvious implications for both identification and treatment of learning disabilities in children and adolescents.

Several definitions of *learning disabilities* exist. The 1987 definition proposed by the National Joint Committee on Learning Disabilities (1987) is frequently cited:

> Learning disabilities is a general term that refers to a heterogeneous group of disorders manifested by significant difficulties in the acquisition and use of listening, speaking, reading, writ-

ing, reasoning, or mathematical abilities. These disorders are intrinsic to the individual, presumed to be due to central nervous system dysfunction, and may occur across the life span. Problems in self-regulatory behaviors, social perception, and social interaction may exist with learning disabilities, but do not by themselves constitute a learning disability. (p. 1)

A more important definition today, however, is the one included in the Individuals With Disabilities Education Act (IDEA; 1997), the federal law that reauthorized and encompassed the Education for All Handicapped Children Act (1975). Under this landmark legislation, all children and youth with disabilities, ages 3–21 years, have the right to a free and appropriate public education. IDEA was subsequently amended with a provision mandating services for infants and toddlers with disabilities and their families. This extended the ages served from birth through 21 years. All states must have a plan that complies with the federal law.

The IDEA defines learning disabilities as

A disorder in one or more of the basic psychological processes involved in understanding or in using language, spoken or written, which may manifest itself in an imperfect ability to listen, read, write, spell, or do mathematical calculations.

Several features of the IDEA have implications specifically for the identification of, assessment of, and services provided for children and adolescents with learning disabilities. Among them are a mandated individualized education program (IEP), some procedural safeguards, and regulations concerning educational placement.

The law, as it pertains to learning disabilities, stipulates that the difficulties in academic skills be the result of "processing disorders" that cause a significant discrepancy between a student's potential and the acquisition of academic skills. IDEA defines *processing* as the sets of mental operations mediated by the central nervous system that access, manipulate, and transform information. These operations include a range of functions that influence the perception, association, storage, and retrieval of information as it is accumulated by the various senses—sight, hearing, and so on. Developmental problems, as other disorders of the central nervous system, may interfere with these operations, resulting in "processing deficits." To be considered learning disabled, both a central processing deficit and the discrepancy criteria must be present.

The extent to which a discrepancy in any given individual is considered significant (i.e., statistically) is open to interpretation (Hallahan and Kauffman 1997; Kavale et al. 1994; B. A. Shaywitz et al. 1992). Under the law, each state is free to establish its own interpretation of the clinical cutoff that defines a processing disorder, as well as its own discrepancy formula. This results in considerable variability from state to state (Coutinho 1995). In addition, to be classified as learning disabled, an individual must have symptoms that meet the DSM-IV criteria (American Psychiatric Association 1994). Although there has been controversy about the inclusion of learning disorders in the classification of mental disorders in DSM-IV, they are similar insofar as they present "a clinically significant behavioral or psychological syndrome or pattern that occurs in an individual and that is associated with present distress...or disability...or with a significantly increased risk of suffering" (American Psychiatric Association 1994, p. xxi).

DSM-IV divides learning disorders into areas of specific academic skills and a not otherwise specified (NOS) category for those not meeting criteria for any specific academic deficit. For designation as learning disabled, an individual's achievement in a particular skill must be substantially below the level of his or her ability as measured and predicated by a standardized IQ test. However, research over the past decade has challenged the advisability of this IQ–achievement discrepancy as a criterion because bright children tend to be overidentified, whereas low achievers are underidentified (Fletcher et al. 1994; S. E. Shaywitz 1996).

Current research supports domain-specific assessment of learning disabilities. This approach promises earlier identification and remediation, in contrast to approaches that are based on the IQ–achievement discrepancy, which require a child to fall behind academically before becoming eligible for treatment.

Learning disorders are diverse in nature and extent and may produce subtle or marked impairments. Some learning disabilities are easily observable on clinical assessment, whereas others are diagnosable only on comprehensive standardized evaluations. Although learning problems for many children are apparent early in life, reading disorders, the most common learning disability, are frequently identified only after the child enters school. Acquired learning disabilities may have their onset at any time (Biederman et al. 1998), resulting from physical trauma, the central nervous system damage of certain infections, or even environmental toxins (Shepherd and Uhry 1993).

Etiology

The specific etiology of learning disabilities usually is difficult to determine, but family, genetic, cognitive, and neuroanatomical factors have been suggested (Hallahan et al. 1996; Love and Webb 1992). The strongest evidence to date supports the heritability of learning disabilities (Pennington 1995). Across family studies, the familial risk to first-degree relatives has been found to be between 35% and 40%, compared with the general population risk of 3%–10%. That is, children of parents with learning disabilities are at least four times more likely to have these problems than children in families without a history of these disorders.

Poor academic performance also may be secondary to emotional problems, psychiatric disorders, or inadequate instruction (Beitchman and Young 1997). Because learning difficulties have multiple etiologies, it is important to define subtypes that reflect the differences that exist among them. These differences may be apparent in etiology, symptoms, and performance, and they also may have implications for treatment. Several subtyping systems have been proposed to identify the distinctive characteristics and antecedents of the various learning disabilities. At present, two general types are commonly recognized: 1) language-based disorders, which are associated primarily with difficulties in reading, spelling, and spoken language, and 2) nonverbal learning disabilities, which affect arithmetic, spatial organization, eye-hand coordination, and, frequently, social-emotional functioning. Unlike the language-based learning disabilities, the nonverbal learning disabilities are associated with the deficits in neurocognitive and adaptive functions that are most often attributed to the right hemisphere of the brain.

Classification

DSM-IV classifies learning disorders on Axis I and categorizes them by specific academic subject area as reading disorder, mathematics disorder, and disorder of written expression. To meet the criteria for a reading disorder, a child's "reading achievement, as measured by individually administered standardized tests of reading accuracy or comprehension," must be "substantially below that expected given the person's chronological age, measured intelligence, and age-appropriate education" (American Psychiatric Association 1994, p. 50). In addition, the disturbance must be sufficiently handicapping to interfere with academic achievement or with the activities of daily life that require reading. If a sensory deficit is present (deafness or visual impairment, for instance), the reading difficulties are in excess of those usually associated with it.

The criteria for mathematics disorder are similar; they test for significant deficits in mathematical ability that impair functioning in school or in the daily activities that require mathematical ability. As in reading, if a sensory deficit is present, the difficulties in mathematics are in excess of those usually associated with it.

For disorder of written expression, the same three criteria must be met for the designation of learning disabled, but this time with the stipulation that the disturbance must interfere with activities "that require the composition of written texts (e.g., writing grammatically correct sentences and organized paragraphs)" (American Psychiatric Association 1994, p. 53).

Learning disorder not otherwise specified covers learning disorders that do not meet the criteria for any specific academic difficulty. Under this diagnosis, any or all of the three subject areas may be affected to a degree that significantly interferes with academic achievement, even if the individual skill does not by itself meet the discrepancy criteria.

Although communication disorders are not included among the DSM-IV learning disorders, delayed or impaired language development is frequently a precursor to later academic and behavioral difficulties (Beitchman et al. 1996). Reading and writing disabilities are most commonly affected by early language disorders (Majsterek and Ellenwood 1995; Torgesen et al. 1994). For example, a young child who has phonological delays, a limited vocabulary, and/or receptive or expressive language disorder is likely to have future difficulties interpreting written symbols and understanding the meaning of print. Similarly, encoding the symbols necessary for written expression and spelling may prove challenging. The data suggest that children with concurrent learning and language disability are at significantly greater risk for a comorbid Axis I disorder (Cantwell and Baker 1991). (Some dyslexic children do have particularly well-developed *oral* language skills, however.)

Epidemiology

Reading disorders are the most commonly identified learning disability. Estimates of their prevalence vary (Kavale and Forness 1995) depending on the assessment procedures and the cutoff points used (B. A. Shaywitz et al. 1992). Although figures range from 2% to 10%, most estimates indicate that about 4% of school-age children and more than 60% of those with a learning disability classification are affected. Although reading disabilities were historically considered discrete disorders (Rutter and Yule 1975), more recent research supports the view that reading problems are found on a normally distributed continuum (B. A. Shaywitz et al. 1992).

Clinical and school-based studies have typically reported significantly higher rates of reading disorders among boys than among girls (Flynn and Rahbar 1994; Shaywitz et al. 1990). Epidemiological studies have found no significant differences between the sexes (Prior et al. 1999; Shaywitz et al. 1990). Boys with reading disabilities are more likely than girls to be noticed in the school setting, however, because of their associated behavioral symptoms. Previously reported differences may be a result of biased referral practices by teachers and the overrepresentation of boys identified. Therefore, it has been suggested that reading-disabled girls need to have serious difficulties before they are referred for diagnosis (Smart et al. 1996).

Nonverbal learning disabilities, which are thought to stem from a disorder in the white matter connections in the right hemisphere of the brain (Cleaver and Whitman 1998; Rourke 1989), occur less frequently than language-based learning disorders. Studies show that among children referred to learning disability clinics, fewer than 10% have nonverbal learning disorders (Denckla 1991; Ingersoll and Goldstein 1993). The presence of nonverbal learning disabilities is sometimes indicated by a significant interscale discrepancy on the Wechsler Intelligence Scale for Children (WISC-III; Wechsler 1991), showing that verbal abilities are clearly superior to performance skills.

The major problems for children with this group of disorders are 1) motoric (lack of coordination, difficulty with handwriting), 2) visual-spatial-organizational (poor visual recall, difficulties with spatial relationships, poor visual-motor coordination), and 3) social (lack of comprehension of nonverbal communication, difficulty adjusting to novel situations, trouble with transitions). Children with nonverbal disabilities, then, are likely to have difficulties with arithmetic and handwriting that may occur with or without associated reading disorders. Deficits in social perception and social judgment are also commonly experienced because nonverbal signals and cues (i.e., body language and facial expressions) are so important in communication.

Rather than improving with age, nonverbal learning disabilities have been shown to worsen over time (Cleaver and Whitman 1998) and to place the individual at risk for social or emotional disturbance, especially anxiety and depression, the internalizing disorders (Beitchman and Young 1997; Casey et al. 1991; Denckla 1991). Girls with mathematics difficulties appear to be at greater risk for adjustment problems than girls with reading problems (Prior et al. 1999).

Diagnosis

The assessment of learning disabilities requires several bases: historical, cognitive, academic, and social. The data in each of these areas are derived from parental and school history, observation of the child, and direct assessment with both informal and standardized measures. Evaluation of cognitive ability (using instruments such as the WISC-III), academic achievement, perceptual and organization skills, and individual learning styles is important to understand the nature of the problem. In addition, examiners must have knowledge of the child's ethnic and cultural environment and the contribution of any relevant psychological factors in order to interpret this information correctly. Too often, the child's motivation and emotional status are not explored in school-based educational evaluations. When a child is referred for assessment, the professionals involved must consider, and try to discern, to what extent learning problems are primary, with secondary effects on the child's mental health, and to what extent primary emotional problems may be affecting his or her academic performance.

For some children and adolescents with learning disabilities, emotional and behavioral issues may be a reflection of a dysfunctional nervous system. Neurobiological study results suggest a continuity between early temperament and later development of psychiatric disorders that may be genetically influenced. Researchers have noted that some infants have difficulty from the earliest stages of development, whereas other learning disabled children and adolescents are unable to move as expected through critical developmental stages (Silver 1998). Parents and pediatricians frequently report that children with learning disabilities have chronic histories, beginning in infancy, of difficulty maintaining neurological equilibrium. The irritability of such infants, and their difficulties in sleeping and eating, although not predictive, seem to presage their future problems.

In a study of preschool children (Thompson and Kronenberger 1990), nonreferred children at risk for developmental and learning problems had higher frequencies of behavior problems than children who were not at risk. Although some children do seem to "outgrow" their difficulties (McGee and Share 1988), many develop low frustration tolerance, explosive outbursts, or aggressive behavior. However, the research suggests that the sense of support and efficacy that good family functioning can provide are protective and reduce the effect of risk.

Social-Emotional Development

The experience of being learning disabled affects psychological development in children and adolescents. Parents and educators have long known that the psychological and social difficulties that characterize children with learning disabilities are often as problematic as the disability itself (Osman 1995). These psychosocial problems further complicate learning, schoolwork, relationships, and the process of development. Learning disabilities adversely affect children's sense of mastery and competence and contribute to the frustration and feelings of inadequacy in those who live and work with the children who have them.

Much has been written in the past decade about the social problems of children and adolescents with learning disabilities (Bender and Wall 1994; Osman 1995). The deficits in cognitive processing that affect learning in academic areas are likely to cause difficulties in other aspects of life as well—for example, in the interpretation of social situations and interpersonal interactions. The ability to function well socially has important implications for a child's self-esteem and for his or her mental health in adolescence and adulthood (Bender and Wall 1994; Mellard and Hazel 1992). It has been well documented that young people with learning disabilities may lack social competence and have difficulty understanding their own or others' affective states, especially in complex or ambiguous situations (Bryan 1991; Osman 1995). Deficits in socially acceptable behavior and social skills, and therefore diminished social acceptance, have been observed in children and adolescents of all ages (Bender and Wall 1994; Osman 1995; Vaughn and LaGreca 1993). Specifically, these children may have more problems in interpersonal relationships and be less accepted socially than their nonhandicapped peers. Research also has shown that some of these deficits may become more acute during the preadolescent and adolescent years (Mellard and Hazel 1992).

The development of social skills within the school setting is an important and salient task for all young people. Studies have reported that students with learning disabilities are rated by teachers, parents, and peers as lacking in social competence as compared with age mates (Bender and Wall 1994; Sabornie 1994; Tur-Kaspa and Bryan 1995). Children with learning disabilities have been found to be less assertive, more dependent, and shy (Wiener et al. 1990) or more aggressive and less cooperative than their nonhandicapped peers, resulting in a lack of acceptance.

The pervasiveness of social difficulties in the learning disorder population became so apparent in the 1980s that the Interagency Committee on Learning Disabilities (ICLD; 1987) recommended that social skills be included in a revised definition of learning disability. This recommendation evoked criticism, however, on the basis that it blurred the boundaries between learning, behavioral, and emotional disorders (Forness and Kavale 1991). In the end, social skills were not included in the federal regulations.

In addition to lacking social acceptance, young people with learning disabilities tend to have low self-esteem and negative attributions for success. They show more external than internal orientations and are likely to perceive social and academic outcomes as being controlled by others or simply by "luck." Moreover, the lower their self-concept, the more likely they are to attribute failure to their inability and incompetence (Cooley and Ayres 1988; Grolnick and Ryan 1990).

After repeated failures, real or imagined, some children develop a sense of what Seligman (1975) has called *learned helplessness*. According to this theory, students develop the perception that outcomes are unrelated to their actions. Thus, they believe that events are uncontrollable, which, in turn, encourages passive or negative behavior. Young people who imagine an external locus of control do not persist in difficult tasks or expect to succeed on future attempts, which bodes ill for achievement. As adolescents, they are afraid to take age-appropriate responsibilities or to venture out on their own. Instead, they remain dependent on adults for decision making and companionship.

Although not coded as Axis I disorders, the consequences of low self-concept and lack of social competence in many children and adolescents with learning disabilities need attention in both research and practice. Increasing evidence indicates that these problems persist over time, leading to adjustment problems, vocational instability, and psychiatric disorders in later life.

Attention-Deficit/Hyperactivity Disorder

The psychiatric disorder most frequently diagnosed in association with learning disabilities is attention-deficit/hyperactivity disorder (ADHD). It is well known that children and adolescents with ADHD tend to underachieve academically; furthermore, underachieving children have significantly increased rates of ADHD. Estimates of the concordance range from 20% to 80% (Hinshaw 1992; Osman 1997; Silver 1998). Although the literature on sustained and selective attention, as well as that on distractibility, in children with learning disabilities clearly demonstrates the overlap (Shaywitz and Shaywitz 1991), the specific nature of the relationship has not been defined.

Some researchers have suggested that inattentiveness, the cardinal construct of ADHD, may be the result of learning difficulties over time (Silver 1998; Weinberg and Emslie 1991), whereas others have hypothesized that the symptoms of ADHD precede and impede academic performance (August and Garfinkel 1990; Smart et al. 1996). It has been shown that early behavioral difficulties, especially those involving deficits in impulse-control and self-regulation skills, predict the development of learning disabilities rather than the reverse (Fergusson and Horwood 1992; Smart et al. 1996). A third view is that ADHD and learning disabilities are separate disorders with a common underlying neurological dysfunction (Spreen 1989) that co-occur in some children (August and Garfinkel 1990; Torgesen 1988).

Neuroimaging studies have found that children with learning disabilities or ADHD do not have the frontal asymmetry typically found in control subjects without these disorders (Hynd et al. 1990; Light et al. 1995). It has also been suggested that because attention and vigilance are functions principally located in the right cerebral hemisphere, the absence of these functions would be consistent with nonverbal (right hemisphere) learning disabilities. Additional research is needed, however, to resolve the question of a shared underlying neurological basis for learning disabilities and ADHD.

Although children with learning disabilities and ADHD have been reported to have problems of attentional performance (August and Garfinkel 1990), some clinicians have found that children with learning disabilities have more difficulty with selective attention, whereas those with ADHD have more problems with sustained attention (Richards et al. 1990). This is controversial, however, because many children and adolescents with learning disabilities and ADHD can selectively sustain their attention to tasks of interest that are within their ability level (Barkley 1990; Osman 1997). Additional investigation is needed with regard to both conditions to formulate appropriate intervention programs for children whose learning disabilities co-occur with ADHD.

Anxiety and Depression

Children and adolescents with learning disabilities frequently react emotionally to their ongoing stress, both intrapersonally and in the school environment. Most young people with learning disabilities are well aware of their deficits from an early age. Even when they possess superior potential, they are likely to become frustrated, knowing that they cannot meet their own standards for achievement or their parents' and teachers' expectations.

The connection between learning disabilities, anxiety, and depression has only recently become a focus of attention in the literature. This may be in part because research has tended to emphasize the reading and language disorders, which are most prevalent. However, the nonverbal (especially mathematical) disabilities are associated with a significantly higher risk for the development of internalized problems, including withdrawal, anxiety and depression, and suicide (Rourke and Fuerst 1992).

Whether learning and internalizing problems (anxiety and depression) are causally connected or merely co-occur is unclear. However, several hypotheses have been suggested (Smart et al. 1996): 1) anxiety and/or depression disrupt the learning process, leading to reading and other disabilities; 2) reading difficulties and the experience of failure engender anxiety and other problems; and 3) common precursors, such as cognitive abilities or social disadvantage, contribute to both learning and internalizing disorders. The possibility of bidirectional paths between both disorders also has been proposed (Hinshaw 1992).

Anxiety is part of the innate human neurobiological system and serves an important protective function, despite its subjective discomfort. It is also a universal experience, inherent in the growth process as children move through early developmental stages into new, more advanced ones. Fears of the dark, of monsters, and of separation from parents are typical in the life of the young child, but over time these normal anxieties generally fade as the child begins to understand the difference between fantasy and reality. Similarly, graduating from school or beginning a new job may provoke anxiety in adolescence but usually is handled without intolerable stress.

Anxiety is considered problematic when it interferes with the normal functioning of the child or adolescent—that is, when it persists beyond normative developmental stages, occurs in inappropriate situations, or becomes overgeneralized. Although some of the research on anxiety strongly suggests the existence of a biological vulnerability in children and adolescents with learning disabilities, learning theorists point to an experiential or learned basis for anxiety. Nonetheless, evidence supports a high rate of familial concordance, whether this occurs by a genetic transmission or as the result of an anxious parenting style.

Children and adolescents with learning disabilities are particularly vulnerable to anxiety disorders, which may be related to genetic endowment, their individual neurobiological systems, immature social or emotional development, or environmental determinants. Empirical research reports higher anxiety levels and lower autonomy levels in both children and adolescents with learning disabilities as compared with their non–learning disabled peers (Stein and Hoover 1989).

From the earliest school years, if not before, children with learning disabilities are likely to experience frustrations in their attempts to learn and stress in the school environment. Some try to avoid the stress, withdrawing to avoid any potentially frustrating or uncertain situation. Others regress to earlier stages of psychological and social development, and their interactions with peers and adults tend to appear immature or infantile as a result (Silver 1993).

An anxious child's symptoms can range from mild restlessness and discomfort to panic attacks. Some children with learning disabilities develop nervous habits or somatic symptoms, and some may be overly concerned about bodily harm or injury. They may be subject to sleep disturbances or eating disorders or be afraid to separate from parents or caregivers. These anxieties tend to escalate over time and may result in symptoms of a generalized anxiety disorder as the child matures into school age. For children and adolescents with learning disabilities, the fear of going to school or doing school assignments and homework can be the catalyst for this disorder.

However, at some point, most children with learning disabilities are likely to feel demoralized or transiently depressed when they compare their accomplishments with those of their peers. Academic failures and poor social interactions typically faced by children with learning disabilities cause them to feel helpless, devalued, and angry. This is almost inherent in the challenge of having a learning disability, but it is not pathological and must be carefully distinguished from childhood depression, which is a clinical disorder with emotional, cognitive, and physical symptoms. Some children become defiant, but others react predominantly with depressed mood or symptoms of clinical depression. Because children and adolescents with learning disabilities are subject to a high risk of stress through the school years, some researchers have suggested that the heightened stress may lead to depression and even suicide (Geisthardt and Munsch 1996; Maag and Reid 1994; McBride and Seigel 1997).

The association of depression with learning disabilities has recently attracted attention in the educational and the psychiatric literature. In part, this reflects the universal concern about the prevalence of depression in children and the increasing number of adolescent suicides. Recognition that even young children can have depressive disorders is now well documented (Ferro et al. 1994; McCauley and Myers 1992).

Most of the research in the area today suggests that children and adolescents with learning disabilities have higher rates of depression than students without these disabilities (Bender and Wall 1994; Mokros et al. 1989; Wright-Strawderman and Watson 1992). Similarly, many children referred for depressive disorders have been found to have cognitive and achievement scores that would qualify them for a learning disorder classification (Weinberg and Emslie 1991). In one study, nearly one of every four depressed or dysthymic children appeared to have a learning disability, suggesting a substantial area of common interest between professionals and parents in both of these areas (Forness and Kavale 1991). It seems likely, therefore, that depression may induce or exacerbate learning difficulties, whereas learning disabilities place children at risk for depression.

Rourke and Fuerst (1992) claimed that nonverbal learning disabilities in particular put children and adolescents at significant risk for depression and possibly even suicide. Cognitive and personality factors such as impulsivity, low self-esteem, and a cognitive weakness in relating cause and effect may increase suicide risk above the risk of depression alone. In other words, some of the very characteristics specifically associated with learning disorders may predispose children and adolescents to suicide (Huntington and Bender et al. 1993; Rourke and Fuerst 1996).

The diagnosis of depression in children is not simple. Although the DSM-IV criteria for depression are the same for children and adults (lethargy, vegetative functions, morbid ideation, and so on), children may tend to express these symptoms differently. Children are much less able to verbalize their feelings than adults, particularly if they have language-based learning disorders. A decline in school performance coupled with social withdrawal, somatic complaints, irritability, or age-inappropriate temper tantrums should alert parents and teachers to the possibility of depression.

However, dysthymia and symptoms of subclinical depression are more common than major depressive disorders among students with learning disabilities. A low level of chronic depression in learning-disabled children may be a psychological response to the perceived disparity between what one "is" and what one "ought to be"; that is, to the loss of the ideal self (Cohen 1985). Children with learning disabilities, especially in highly educated or achievement-oriented families, may feel inadequate for having failed to satisfy their (or their parents') ego ideal.

The child's history as given by parents and by the school can help to differentiate a primary depression with cognitive effects from depressive feelings secondary to learning difficulties, but confusion of symptom and syndrome is not uncommon in children and adolescents with learning disabilities and depression. The consequences of depression are so serious, however, that professionals must be extremely alert to signs of either and must make every effort to diagnose the situation accurately and address it comprehensively.

Acting-Out Behaviors

Some children and adolescents with learning disabilities internalize their problems, but others externalize them, becoming so frustrated and angry over their learning, social, and family difficulties that they act out their frustrations and emotional conflicts. They misbehave, disrupt the classroom, and get into conflicts with teachers, parents, and peers. A child often may appear initially as anxious or depressed, may appear later as oppositional and defiant, and finally may act in adolescence in ways that meet the criteria for a conduct disorder.

Children with disruptive behavior disorders are more likely than anxious or depressed children to be identified in school (Hinshaw 1992; Sanson et al. 1996). A high incidence of aggressive and antisocial behaviors have been reported in children with learning disabilities. However, behavior problems in children and adolescents with learning disabilities *are not necessarily an indication of emotional disorders.* These behaviors may be part of the underlying neurodevelopmental delays associated with the learning disabilities. Cognitive deficits and speech or language problems have been shown to be risk factors for conduct disorders (Benasich et al. 1993; Cantwell and Baker 1991; Hinshaw 1992). Whether the accompanying deficits in academic performance represent antecedents or consequences of the disorder is unclear (Hinshaw 1992).

Indications are, however, that moderate to severe behavior problems at any age persist unless treated (Benasich et al. 1993). They set in motion a series of ongoing psychological processes that are destructive to the development of the child and frequently to society as well. Adolescents with unremediated learning disabilities appear to be particularly vulnerable to drug and alcohol abuse as well as to behaviors that violate the rights of others. They are more likely to leave school prematurely and to have vocational difficulties as a result of their educational disadvantage. Preventive interventions clearly are needed to reduce the number of risk factors for learning disabilities in children and to increase the number of protective factors in their environment.

Treatment

Effective treatment and support for children with learning disabilities are especially important when their problems are viewed from a long-term perspective. It is well known that these learning disorders are persistent and increase the risk of being held back in school, dropping out prematurely, and developing co-occurring personality and emotional disorders (Spreen 1989). The risks are further elevated when a disadvantaged background is factored in.

The keystone of intervention for children and adolescents is the provision within the school of special education services, as mandated by law. Today, most children with learning disabilities are educated in general education classes, which are considered to be "the least restrictive environment" (IDEA), with additional supports (Zigmond 1995). Whereas in the past, approaches to remediation focused on underlying academic deficits, efforts now are centered on direct instruction of component skills. An important corollary for successful outcomes is an accurate assessment of the severity of the learning disabilities and the contexts in which they arise.

Current wisdom dictates that whenever a concurrent behavioral or emotional disorder is contributing to academic underachievement, intervention is warranted. Recent findings regarding the sequelae of learning disabilities emphasize the importance of comprehensive multidisciplinary assessment and follow-up of children at risk. If treatment for comorbid disorders is indicated, the clinician can be pivotal in helping the child and family address the problems.

Multimodal treatment based on assessment of all clinical factors has been shown to improve children's academic, behavioral, and emotional adjustment (Hammill 1990; Osman 1997; Silver 1993). Direct treatment is warranted for concurrent psychiatric and other secondary emotional and social problems (Forness and Kavale

1996; Kauffman 1997). Individual, family, and/or group psychotherapy may be recommended, and medical intervention may be indicated. However, any psychotherapeutic approach must be tailored to the child's specific learning disabilities. For the child with language problems, interventions that include nonverbal approaches (e.g., games and computers) are likely to have better results than an exclusively language-based treatment. Mental health professionals must understand the learning disabled child's underlying neurological difficulties and the effects that these have on his or her social development. The clinician also must be aware to what extent the learning disabilities may interfere with the therapeutic process and make the necessary adaptations (Silver 1993).

Because attention-deficit disorders and learning disabilities co-occur frequently, the use of stimulant medications is common. Improvement in attention and concentration can help the child participate in the learning environment and lead to an increase in work completed (Osman 1999). However, the possible side effects, such as decreased appetite and insomnia, as well as the therapeutic benefits, must be considered. The efficacy of psychopharmacological intervention for learning disabilities alone in the absence of ADHD, however, is questionable, unless, of course, comorbid psychiatric symptoms must be addressed.

Today, increasing numbers of psychotropic medications are used for children and adolescents, with positive results. They should not be used in isolation, however, but rather as part of a coordinated treatment plan. Psychiatrists, psychopharmacologists, and other mental health professionals should contribute their particular skills and expertise to provide the appropriate treatment for any given child. Moreover, they also may have to assume an educational role while treating learning disabilities in children and adolescents (Forness and Kavale 1989). In collaboration with school personnel, they are frequently the professionals who can help parents, and perhaps most important, the young people themselves understand the nature of their disorders and their own characteristic styles of coping (Osman 1997).

Whatever approaches to treatment are adopted, the most positive outcomes for children and adolescents with learning disabilities have consistently emerged from studies in which the children received specialized attention at school, support at home, and mental health services when warranted. Young people with learning disabilities represent a diverse group with a broad range of needs. To serve them appropriately and effectively, educational services and clinical care must be coordinated and individualized. The need for interaction between family, school personnel, and physicians is no different from that for children with other medical problems. The aim in all cases is to provide interventions that are realistic and beneficial to the child, the family, and the school.

References

American Psychiatric Association: Diagnostic and Statistical Manual of Mental Disorders, 4th Edition. Washington, DC, American Psychiatric Association, 1994

August GJ, Garfinkel BD: Comorbidity of ADHD among clinic referred children. J Abnormal Psychol 18:29–45, 1990

Barkley RA: Attention Deficit Hyperactivity Disorder. New York, Guilford, 1990

Beitchman JH, Young A: Learning disorders with a special emphasis on reading disorders: a review of the past 10 years. J Am Acad Child Adolesc Psychiatry 36:1020–1032, 1997

Beitchman JH, Wilson B, Brownlie EB, et al: Long-term consistency in speech/language profiles, I: developmental and academic outcomes. J Am Acad Child Adolesc Psychiatry 35:1–11, 1996

Benasich AA, Curtiss S, Tallal P: Language, learning, and behavioral disturbances in childhood: a longitudinal perspective. J Am Acad Child Adolesc Psychiatry 32:585–594, 1993

Bender WN, Wall ME: Social-emotional development of students with learning disabilities. Learning Disabilities Quarterly 17:323–341, 1994

Biederman JH, Cantwell DP, Forness SR, et al: Practice parameters for the assessment and treatment of children and adolescents with language and learning disorders. J Am Acad Child Adolesc Psychiatry 37 (10, suppl):46S–62S, 1998

Boetsch E, Green PA, Pennington BF: Psychosocial correlates of dyslexia across the life span. Dev Psychopathol 8:539–562, 1996

Bryan T: Social problems and learning disabilities, in Learning About Learning Disabilities. Edited by Wong BY. San Diego, CA, Academic Press, 1991, pp 195–229

Butkowsky IS, Willows DM: Cognitive-motivational characteristics of children varying in reading ability: evidence for learned helplessness in poor readers. J Educ Psychol 72:408–422, 1980

Cantwell DP, Baker I: Psychiatric and Developmental Disorders in Children With Communication Disorder. Washington, DC, American Psychiatric Press, 1991

Casey JE, Rourke BP, Picard EM: Syndrome of nonverbal learning disabilities: age differences in neuropsychological, academic, and socioemotional functioning. Dev Psychopathol 3:329–345, 1991

Cleaver RL, Whitman RD: Right hemisphere, white matter learning disabilities associated with depression in an adolescent and young adult psychiatric population. J Nerv Ment Dis 186:561–565, 1998

Cohen J: Learning disabilities and adolescence: developmental considerations, in Adolescent Psychiatry: Developmental and Clinical Studies, Vol 12. Chicago, IL, University of Chicago, 1985

Cohen NJ, Davine M, Horodesky N, et al: Unsuspected language impairments in psychiatrically disturbed children: prevalence and language and behavioral characteristics. J Am Acad Child Adolesc Psychiatry 32:595–603, 1993

Cooley EJ, Ayres RR: Self-concept and success-failure attributions of nonhandicapped students with learning disabilities. J Learn Disabil 21:174–178, 1988

Coutinho MJ: Who will be learning disabled after the reauthorization of IDEA? Two very distinct perspectives. J Learn Disabil 28:664–671,1995

Denckla MB: Academic and extracurricular aspects of nonverbal learning disabilities. Psychiatric Annals 21:717–724, 1991

Fergusson DM, Horwood IJ: Attention deficit and reading achievement. J Child Psychol Psychiatry 33:375–385, 1992

Fergusson DM, Lynskey MT: Early reading problems and later conduct problems. J Child Psychol Psychiatry 33:899–907, 1997

Ferro T, Carlson GA, Grayson P, et al: Depressive disorders: distinctions in children. J Am Acad Child Adolesc Psychiatry 33:664–670, 1994

Fletcher JM, Shaywitz SE, Shankweiler DP, et al: Cognitive profiles of reading disability: comparisons of discrepancy and low achievement definitions. J Educ Psychol 86:6–23, 1994

Flynn JM, Rahbar MH: Prevalence of reading failure in boys compared with girls. Psychology in the Schools 331:66–71, 1994

Forness SR, Kavale KA: Identification and diagnostic issues in special education: a status report for child psychiatrists. Child Psychiatry Hum Dev 19:279–301, 1989

Forness SR, Kavale KA: Social skills deficits as primary learning disabilities: a note on problems with the ICLD diagnostic criteria. Learning Disabilities: Research and Practice 6:44–49, 1991

Forness SR, Kavale KA: Treating social skills deficits in children with learning disabilities: a meta-analysis. Learning Disabilities Quarterly 19:80–89, 1996

Geisthardt C, Munsch J: Coping with school stress: a comparison of adolescents with and without learning disabilities. J Learn Disabil 29:287–296, 1996

Grolnick WS, Ryan RM: Self-perceptions, motivation, and adjustment in children with learning disabilities: a multiple group comparison study. J Learn Disabil 23:177–184, 1990

Hallahan DP, Kauffman JM: Exceptional Learners: Introduction to Special Education, 7th Edition. Boston, MA, Allyn & Bacon, 1997

Hallahan DP, Kauffman JM, Lloyd JW: Introduction to Learning Disabilities, 3rd Edition. Englewood Cliffs, NJ, Prentice-Hall, 1996

Hammill DD: On defining learning disabilities: an emerging consensus. J Learn Disabil 23:74–84, 1990

Hinshaw SP: Externalizing behavior problems and academic underachievement in childhood and adolescence: causal relationships and underlying mechanisms. Psychol Bull 111:127–155, 1992

Huntington DD, Bender WN: Adolescents with learning disabilities at risk? Emotional well-being, depression, suicide. J Learn Disabil 26:159–166, 1993

Hynd GW, Semrud-Clikeman M, Lorys AR, et al: Brain morphology in developmental dyslexia and attention deficit disorder/hyperactivity. Arch Neurol 47:919–926, 1990

Individuals With Disabilities Education Act (IDEA), PL 105–17 SEC 601 [20 USC 1400], 1997

Ingersoll BD, Goldstein S: Attention Deficit Disorder and Learning Disabilities. New York, Doubleday, 1993

Kauffman JM: Characteristics of Emotional and Behavioral Disorders of Children and Youth, 6th Edition. Englewood Cliffs, NJ, Prentice-Hall, 1997

Kavale KA, Forness SR: The Nature of Learning Disabilities: Critical Elements of Diagnosis and Classification. Matawa, NJ, Lawrence Erlbaum, 1995

Kavale KA, Fuchs D, Scruggs TE: Setting the record straight on learning disability and low achievement: implications for policy making. Learning Disabilities: Research and Practice 9:70–77, 1994

Light JG, Pennington BF, Gilger JW, et al: Reading disability and hyperactivity disorder: evidence for a common genetic etiology. Developmental Neuropsychiatry 11:323–335, 1995

Little SS: Nonverbal learning disabilities and socioemotional functioning: a review of recent literature. J Learn Disabil 26:653–655, 1993

Love R, Webb W: Neurology for the Speech-Language Pathologist. Boston, MA, Butterworth-Heinemann, 1992

Maag HW, Reid R: The phenomenology of depression among students with and without learning disabilities: more similar than different. Learning Disabilities: Research and Practice 9:91–103, 1994

Majsterek DJ, Ellenwood AE: Phonological awareness and beginning reading: evaluation of a school-based screening procedure. J Learn Disabil 28:449–456, 1995

McBride HEA, Seigel LS: Learning disabilities and adolescent suicide. J Learn Disabil 30:652–659, 1997

McCauley E, Myers K: The longitudinal and clinical course of depression in children and adolescents. Child and Adolescent Psychiatric Clinics of North America 1(1):183–196, 1992

McGee R, Share DL: Attention deficit disorder–hyperactivity and academic failure: which comes first and what should be treated? J Am Acad Child Adolesc Psychiatry 27:318–325, 1988

Mellard DF, Hazel JS: Social competencies as a pathway to successful life transitions. Learning Disabilities Quarterly 15:251–271, 1992

Mokros HB, Poznanski EO, Merrick WA: Depression and learning disabilities in children: a test of an hypothesis. J Learn Disabil 22:230–233, 244, 1989

National Joint Committee on Learning Disabilities Interagency Committee on Learning Disabilities: Learning Disabilities: A Report to the U.S. Congress. Bethesda, MD, National Institutes of Health, 1987

Osman B: No One to Play With: Social Problems of LD and ADD Children. Novato, CA, Academic Therapy Publications, 1995

Osman BB: Learning Disabilities and ADHD: A Family Guide to Living and Learning Together. New York, John Wiley & Sons, 1997

Osman BB: Coordinating care in the prescription and use of Ritalin with ADHD children and adolescents, in Ritalin: Theory and Practice. Edited by Greenhill LL, Osman BB. New York, Mary Ann Liebert, 1999, pp 175–193

Pennington BF: Genetics of learning disabilities. J Child Neurol 10 (suppl 1):S69–S77, 1995

Prior M: Understanding Specific Learning Disabilities. Sussex, England, Psychology Press, 1996

Prior M, Smart D, Sanson A, et al: Relationships between learning difficulties and psychological problems in preadolescent children from a longitudinal sample. Journal of Child and Adolescent Psychiatry 38:429–436, 1999

Richards GP, Samuels SJ, Turnure JE, et al: Sustained and selective attention in children with learning disabilities. J Learn Disabil 23:129–136, 1990

Rothstein LF: Special Education Law. New York, Longman, 1990

Rourke BP: Nonverbal Learning Disabilities: The Syndrome and the Model. New York, Guilford, 1989

Rourke BP, Fuerst DR: Socioemotional disturbances of learning disabled children. J Consult Clin Psychol 56:801–810, 1992

Rourke BP, Fuerst DR: Psychological dimensions of learning disability subtypes. Assessment 3:277–290, 1996

Rutter M, Yule W: The concept of specific reading retardation. J Child Psychol Psychiatry 16:181–197, 1975

Sabornie EJ: Social-affective characteristics in early adolescents identified as learning disabled and nondisabled. Learning Disability Quarterly 17:268–279, 1994

Sanson A Prior M, Smart D: Predicting reading difficulties and behavioral problems at 7–8 years from longitudinal data from infancy to 6 years. J Child Psychol Psychiatry 37:529–541, 1996

Seligman MEP: Helplessness: On Depression, Development, and Death. San Francisco, CA, Freeman, 1975

Shaywitz BA, Shaywitz SE: Comorbidity: a critical issue in attention deficit disorder. J Child Neurol 6:S13–S22, 1991

Shaywitz BA, Fletcher J, Holahan JM, et al: Discrepancy compared to low achievement definitions of reading disability: results from the Connecticut Longitudinal Study. J Learn Disabil 25:639–648, 1992

Shaywitz SE, Shaywitz BA, Fletcher JM, et al: Prevalence of reading difficulty in boys and girls: results of the Connecticut Longitudinal Study. JAMA 264:998–1000, 1990

Shaywitz SE, Fletcher JM, Shaywitz BA: A conceptual model and definition of dyslexia: findings emerging from the Connecticut Longitudinal Study, in Language, Learning, and Behavior Disorders: Developmental, Biological and Clinical Perspectives. Edited by Beitchman J, Cohen N, Konstantareas M, et al. New York, Cambridge University Press, 1996, pp 199–223

Shepherd MJ, Uhry JK: Reading disorder. Child and Adolescent Psychiatric Clinics of North America 2:193–208, 1993

Silver LB: The secondary emotional, social, and family problems found with children and adolescents with learning disabilities. Child and Adolescent Pediatric Clinics of North America 2:295–308, 1993

Silver LB: The Misunderstood Child: Understanding and Coping With Your Child's Learning Disabilities. New York, Times Books, 1998

Smart D, Sanson A, Prior M: Connections between reading disability and behavior problems: testing temporal and causal hypotheses. J Abnorm Child Psychol 24:363–383, 1996

Spreen O: Relationship between learning disability, emotional disorders, and neuropsychology: some results and observations. J Clin Exp Neuropsychol 11:117–140, 1989

Stein PA, Hoover JH: Manifest anxiety in children with learning disabilities. J Learn Disabil 22:66–71, 1989

Torgesen JK: The cognitive and behavioral characteristics of children with learning disabilities. J Learn Disabil 21:341–345, 1988

Torgesen J, Wagner RK, Rashotte CA: Longitudinal studies of phonological processing and reading. J Learn Disabil 27:276–286, 1994

Tur-Kaspa H, Bryan T: Teachers' ratings of the social competence and school adjustment of students with LD in elementary and junior high school. J Learn Disabil 28:44–52, 1995

Vaughn S, LaGreca A: Social skills training: why, who, what and how, in Learning Disabilities: Best Practices for Professionals. Edited by Bender WN. Boston, MA, Andover Medical Publishers, 1993, pp 177–184, 251–273

Wechsler D: Wechsler Intelligence Scale for Children, 3rd Edition (WISC-III). New York, Psychological Corporation, 1991

Weinberg WA, Emslie GJ: Attention deficit hyperactivity disorder in children: a neglected syndrome? J Child Neurol 6 (suppl):S23–S37, 1991

Wiener J, Harris PJ, Shirer C: Achievement and social-behavioral correlates of peer status in LD children. Learning Disability Quarterly 13:114–127, 1990

Wright-Strawderman C, Watson BL: The prevalence of depressive symptoms in children with learning disabilities. J Learn Disabil 25:258–264, 1992

Zigmond N: Models for delivery of special education with learning disabilities in public schools. J Child Neurol 10 (suppl):586–592, 1995

Chapter 3

What Cognitive and Neurobiological Studies Have Taught Us About Dyslexia

Bennett A. Shaywitz, M.D.
Kenneth R. Pugh, Ph.D.
Jack M. Fletcher, Ph.D.
Sally E. Shaywitz, M.D.

Developmental dyslexia is characterized by an unexpected difficulty in reading in children and adults who otherwise have the intelligence, motivation, and schooling considered necessary for accurate and fluent reading. Dyslexia (or specific reading disability) is the most common and most carefully studied of the learning disabilities and affects 80% of all individuals identified as learning disabled (Lerner 1989). Although in the past the diagnosis and implications of dyslexia often were uncertain, recent advances in our knowledge of the epidemiology, the cognitive influences, the genetics, and the neurobiology now allow the disorder to be approached within a more secure framework. In this chapter, we focus on the cognitive and neurobiological advances in dyslexia and their

Portions of this chapter are substantially similar to other works by us that appeared in Shaywitz BA, Shaywitz SE, Pugh KR, et al.: "The Functional Organization of Brain for Reading and Reading Disability (Dyslexia)." *The Neuroscientist* 2:245–255, 1996; Shaywitz SE, Shaywitz BA: "Dyslexia," in *Pediatric Neurology*. Edited by Swaiman K (in press); Shaywitz BA, Pugh KR, Jenner AR, et al.: "The Neurobiology of Reading and Reading Disability (Dyslexia)," in *Handbook of Reading Research*, Vol. III. Edited by Kamil ML, Mosenthal PB, Pearson PD, et al. Mahwah, NJ, Lawrence Erlbaum (in press); Shaywitz SE: "Current Concepts: Dyslexia." *New England Journal of Medicine* 338:307–312, 1998.

clinical implications for children and, particularly, young adults with this most common and often underrecognized disorder. The reader is referred elsewhere for information about the history, etiology, and genetics of the disorder (S. E. Shaywitz 1996, 1998).

Epidemiology of Dyslexia

Recent epidemiological data indicate that, like hypertension, dyslexia fits a dimensional model. In other words, within the population, reading and reading disability occur along a continuum, with reading disability representing the lower tail of a normal distribution of reading ability (Gilger et al. 1996; S. E. Shaywitz et al. 1992). Dyslexia is perhaps the most common neurobehavioral disorder affecting children, with prevalence rates varying from 5%–10% (Interagency Committee on Learning Disabilities 1987) to 17.5% (S. E. Shaywitz et al. 1994).

Previously, it was believed that dyslexia affected primarily males (Finucci and Childs 1981); however, more recent data (Flynn and Rahbar 1994; S. E. Shaywitz et al. 1990; Wadsworth et al. 1992) indicate comparable numbers of affected males and females. Data derived from the Connecticut Longitudinal Study (S. E. Shaywitz et al. 1990) provided evidence that the presumed increase in prevalence in males found in some studies may reflect sampling bias. This study was based on a sample survey of Connecticut schoolchildren followed longitudinally from kindergarten to third grade and is unique in that all 445 children in the sample received complete ability and reading achievement tests. In this population-based study, numbers of reading-disabled males (8.7%) and females (6.9%) were comparable. Sampling bias inherent in school identification procedures may result in reports of an increased prevalence of reading disability in males in school-identified samples. In contrast, when results are based on test scores in studies in which all children in a population are individually tested, no significant differences in prevalence between males and females are observed.

Longitudinal studies, both prospective (Francis et al. 1996; B. A. Shaywitz et al. 1995c) and retrospective (Bruck 1992; Felton et al. 1990; Scarborough 1984), indicate that dyslexia is a persistent, chronic condition; it does not represent a transient "developmental lag." Over time, poor readers and good readers tend to maintain their relative positions along the reading spectrum (B. A. Shaywitz et al. 1995a).

Cognitive Basis of Dyslexia

Reading, the process of extracting meaning from print, involves both visual-perceptual and linguistic processes. Theories of dyslexia based on the visual system (Stein 1993; Stein and Walsh 1997), on the language system (Shankweiler et al. 1979), on the cerebellum (Nicolson et al. 1995), and on other factors such as temporal processing of stimuli within these systems (Stein and Walsh 1997; Tallal and Stark 1982) have each been proposed. Whatever the contributions of other systems and processes, the current strong consensus among investigators in the field is that the core difficulty in dyslexia reflects a deficiency within the language system.

The evidence that writing systems are, in fact, "merely a way of recording language by visible marks" (Bloomfield 1933, p. 21) seems incontrovertible. In essence, both reading and writing represent the language system. To understand reading, one must first understand the language system and, in particular, the relation between language and reading. Language is served by specific neural systems, an apparatus or language module that evolved in humans and first allowed the emergence of speech some 100,000 to several million years ago (Pinker 1991). Within a modular framework, the language system is conceptualized as a hierarchical series of components: at higher levels are neural systems engaged in processing, for example, semantics, syntax, and discourse; at the lowest level is the phonological module dedicated to processing the distinctive sound elements that constitute language. The functional unit of the phonological module is the phoneme, defined as the smallest discernible segment of speech. Phonemes serve as the basic building blocks of all spoken and written language. For example, the word *bat* is composed of three separate phonemes: buh, aah, tuh.

Within this context, it may be helpful to recall that written language is considered a communication system based on two essential features: 1) phonemes, representing the basic linguistic units, and 2) symbols or written elements used to represent the inventory of phonemes. In the English language, letters of the alphabet serve this symbolic function, so that the 26 letters of the alphabet, singly or in combination, represent the 44 phonemes composing the language. On a representational level, these letter groupings, or graphemes, serve as the written proxys for phonemes and thus function as the operational units of our writing system. Consequently, in addition to developing an awareness of the segmental nature of speech, the beginning reader must come to the realization that written words, too, have an internal phonological structure, that the orthography represents this sound structure, and that the printed word is represented by the same underlying sound or phonological structure as the spoken word.

Phonemes and their graphic symbols thus represent the functional units of language, both spoken and written. In speaking, the phonological units are coarticulated, that is, they are automatically merged and blended, so that there is no overt clue to the underlying segmental nature of speech, and, as a result, spoken language appears seamless. But the phonological specialization performs both speech and listening effortlessly, automatically coarticulating the phonological gestures for the speaker, while also carrying out the reverse process for the listener—that is, automatically parsing or segmenting the coarticulated utterances into their underlying phonological elements. This is no mean feat, for during normal speech, 10–12 phonemes are presented each second, and during rapid speech, this may rise to 25 phonemes/second. The language apparatus assembles the phonology for the speaker and recovers the phonology for the listener. Because both the coarticulation and the parsing functions are performed automatically and unconsciously for speaker and listener, respectively, neither has to develop an awareness of the basic sound structure of language.

Now we can understand the task facing the beginning reader. Speaking is automatic but reading is not. To read, one must realize that the orthography is related to and, indeed, represents the phonology of spoken language; that is, the reader must enter the language system. Operationally, this means that the reader must develop an awareness of the internal phonological structure of words and discover that the orthography represents this basic sound structure. This awareness allows the reader to connect the letter strings (the orthography) to the corresponding units of speech (phonological constituents) they represent. As numerous studies have shown, however, such awareness is largely missing in dyslexic children and adults (Brady and Shankweiler 1991; Bruck 1992; Fletcher et al. 1994; Rieben and Perfetti 1991; Shankweiler et al. 1995; Stanovich and Siegel 1994). As for why dyslexic readers should have exceptional difficulty developing phonological awareness, there is support for the notion that the difficulty resides in the phonological component of the larger specialization for language (A. M. Liberman 1996, 1998; I. Y. Liberman et al. 1989). If that component is imperfect, its representations will be less than ideally distinct and therefore harder to bring to conscious awareness. Now overwhelming evidence indicates that phonological awareness is characteristically deficient in dyslexic readers who, therefore, have difficulty mapping the alphabetic characters onto the spoken word. Abundant evidence relates a deficit in phonological analysis to difficulties in learning to read: phonological measures predict later reading achievement (Bradley and Bryant 1983; Stanovich et al. 1984; Torgesen et al. 1994); deficits in phonological awareness (i.e., awareness that words can be broken down into smaller segments of sound) consistently separate dyslexic and nondisabled children (Fletcher et al. 1994; Stanovich and Siegel 1994); phonological deficits persist into adulthood (Bruck 1992; Felton et al. 1990); and instruction in phonological awareness promotes the acquisition of reading skills (Ball and Blachman 1991; Bradley and Bryant 1983; Foorman et al. 1997; Torgesen et al. 1992; B. W. Wise and Olson 1995). Additional findings of strong heritability for phonological awareness suggest "that it may be the main proximal cause of most genetically-based deficits in word recognition, and thus it may be the most appropriate focus for diagnosis and remediation" (Olson et al. 1994, p. 61).

Neural Basis for Dyslexia

With the elucidation of the cognitive deficit in dyslexia, the stage was set to delineate the neural mechanisms underlying the deficit in phonological analysis. In the next section, we review the evidence that now allows investigators to begin to understand the neurobiological underpinnings of dyslexia. We have chosen to emphasize functional imaging studies, that is, those studies directed at understanding the functional organization of the brain as dyslexic readers engage in tasks tapping the component processes of reading.

Neuroanatomical and Morphometric Studies in Dyslexia

Only in recent years have systematic neuroanatomical studies, which used postmortem anatomical measures and structural morphometric techniques, attempted to relate abnormalities in brain structure to reading and dyslexia (Galaburda and Kemper 1979; Galaburda et al. 1985; Humphreys et al. 1990). Significant methodological limitations (Hynd and Semrud-Clikeman 1989) are imposed on such postmortem studies, but fortunately the development of neuroimaging procedures offers an attractive alternative strategy with which to examine neuroanatomical correlates of dyslexia. Early computed tomography (CT) studies seemed to confirm a reversed or lack of the normal asymmetry in dyslexic individuals (Hier et al. 1978; Leisman and Ashkenazi 1980; LeMay 1981; Rosenberger and Hier 1980), but later reports failed to confirm any differences (Denckla et al. 1985; Haslam et al. 1981; Parkins et al. 1987; Rumsey et al. 1986). More recent magnetic resonance imaging (MRI) reports have not clarified the controversy (Duara et al. 1991; Hynd et al. 1990; Jernigan et al. 1991; Larsen et al. 1990; Leonard et al. 1993) (Table 3–1). Review of these previous studies indicates wide variations in subjects' age, sex, and handedness and in the diagnostic criteria used to define dyslexia. Lack of consistent results among studies might be explained by these factors.

Much has been learned from studies of cerebral localization of cognitive function based on studies of individuals with brain damage, and such studies continue to provide important information, particularly with the emergence of modern imaging methods that allow very fine-grained anatomical resolution (Damasio and

Table 3–1. Tasks and subtractions

Task	Stimuli	Processes engaged
Line	/ / \ / / / \ /	Visuospatial
Case	bbBb	Visuospatial + orthographic
Single-letter rhyme	T V	Visuospatial + orthographic + phonological
Nonword rhyme	LEAT JETE	Visuospatial + orthographic + phonological
Category	CORN	Visuospatial + orthographic + phonological + semantic

Subtractions		Processes isolated
Case–line		Orthographic
Rhyme–line		Orthographic + phonological
Rhyme–case		Phonological
Category–line		Orthographic + phonological + semantic
Category–rhyme		Semantic
Category–case		Phonological + semantic

Damasio 1992). However, studies localizing cerebral function with morphometric measures provide a static picture of brain anatomy rather than a dynamic view of brain function while individuals are performing a cognitive task. The ability to image and then to identify the functional units of the working nervous system, the neural networks that are engaged by specific cognitive functions, is necessary.

Functional imaging, the ability to measure brain function during performance of a cognitive task, meets such a requirement and became possible in the early 1980s. For the first time, rather than being limited to examining the brain in an autopsy specimen, or measuring the size of brain regions with static morphometric indices based on CT or MRI, scientists were able to think of studying brain metabolism while individuals were performing specific cognitive tasks.

Functional Brain Imaging

One approach uses electrophysiological methods (e.g., event-related potentials). Older studies were detailed by Hughes (1977), and more recent ones were reviewed by Dool et al. (1993). Methodological reviews of progress and newer electrographic technologies are provided in reviews by Swick et al. (1994), Thatcher (1996), and Wood et al. (1996). A recent study of this kind (Salmelin et al. 1996) used magnetoencephalography and found that in contrast to nonimpaired readers, dyslexic readers failed to activate the left inferior temporo-occipital region (including Wernicke's area) while reading real words.

General principles of functional brain imaging. Although magnetoencephalography is useful for determining the time course of cognitive processes, it is not nearly as precise as the imaging modalities for localizing where in the brain these processes occur. In principle, functional imaging is quite simple. When an individual is asked to perform a discrete cognitive task, that task places processing demands on particular neural systems in the brain. To meet those demands requires activation of neural systems in specific brain regions, and those changes in neural activity are reflected by changes in brain metabolic activity, which, in turn, are reflected by cerebral blood flow and in the cerebral use of metabolic substrates such as glucose. Functional imaging makes it possible to measure those changes in metabolic activity and blood flow in specific brain regions while subjects are engaged in cognitive tasks.

Xenon and positron-emission tomography. The first studies of this kind used xenon 133 single photon emission computed tomography (SPECT) to measure cerebral blood flow at baseline rather than during any reading task (Flowers et al. 1991; Lou et al. 1984, 1990; Wood et al. 1991). Several studies have used positron-emission tomography (PET). In practice, PET requires intra-arterial or intravenous administration of a radioactive isotope so that either cerebral blood flow using oxygen 15 (^{15}O) or cerebral utilization of glucose using fluorine 18 (^{18}F) fluorodeoxyglucose (FDG) can be determined while the subject is performing a task. Positron-emitting isotopes of nuclei of biological interest have very short biological half-lives and are synthesized in a cyclotron immediately prior to testing, a factor that mandates that the time course of the experiment conform to the short half-life of the radioisotope.

Rumsey et al. (1992) used PET and measured cerebral blood flow using ^{15}O in dyslexic readers listening to determine whether real words rhymed. Dyslexic readers failed to activate the left parietal and left middle temporal regions. In a second report, Rumsey et al. (1994) again used ^{15}O PET during a semantic judgment: that is, to determine whether the meaning of two sentence pairs was the same. Both nonimpaired and dyslexic readers increased cerebral blood flow in the middle temporal regions during the task; no significant differences were observed between nonimpaired and dyslexic readers.

Paulesu et al. (1996) used ^{15}O PET to compare university students with histories of reading problems but who were currently reading in the average range with similarly aged subjects without histories of reading problems; one task required subjects to rhyme single letters, and a companion task involved short-term memory for single letters. Dyslexic readers activated Broca's area during the single-letter rhyme task and Wernicke's area during the memory task, but, in contrast to control subjects, both language regions were not activated in concert in either task. The authors attributed the problem to a disconnection between the anterior and posterior language regions, a theory supported by their finding of underactivation in the insula in this group of dyslexic adults.

In a recent report, Rumsey et al. (1997) used ^{15}O PET to study dyslexic men while they performed two pronunciation tasks (low-frequency real words and pseudowords) and two lexical decision tasks (orthographic and phonological). Compared with control subjects, dyslexic readers had reduced blood flow in the temporal cortex and inferior parietal cortex, especially on the left, during both pronunciation and decision making.

Functional magnetic resonance imaging. Functional magnetic resonance imaging (fMRI) promises to surpass other methods for its ability to map the individual brain's response to specific cognitive stimuli. Because it is noninvasive and safe, it can be used repeatedly, properties that make it ideal for human cognitive studies, especially in children. In principle, the signal used to construct MRIs changes, by a small amount (typically on the order of 1%–5%), in regions that are activated by a stimulus or task. The increase in signal results from the combined effects of increases in the tissue blood flow, volume, and oxygenation, although the precise contributions of each of these are still somewhat uncertain. MRI intensity increases when deoxygenated blood is replaced by oxygenated blood. Various methods can be used to record the changes that occur, but one preferred approach makes use of ultrafast imaging, such as echo planar imaging, in which complete images are acquired in times substantially shorter than a second. Echo planar imaging can provide images at a rate fast enough to capture the time course of the hemodynamic response to neural activation and to permit a wide variety of imaging paradigms over large volumes of the brain. Details of fMRI are reviewed in Anderson and Gore (1997).

Recent progress using fMRI to study reading.   Most functional imaging studies, whether PET or fMRI, use a subtraction methodology in attempting to isolate brain and cognitive function relations (Friston et al. 1993; Sergent 1994). Reading can be considered as involving three component processes: orthographic, phonological, and lexical semantic processing. Accordingly, the tasks should be able to isolate orthographic, phonological, and lexical semantic foci. In addition, we use a variety of subtractions in order to converge on a conclusion about the relative function of a given cortical region.

A typical series of tasks is illustrated in Table 3–1. Both the decision and the response components of the tasks are comparable; in each instance, the subject views two simultaneously presented stimulus displays, one above the other, and is asked to judge them as the same or different by pressing a response button if the displays match on a given cognitive dimension: line orientation judgment, letter case judgment, single-letter rhyme, nonword rhyme, and category judgment. The five tasks are ordered hierarchically:

1. The line orientation judgment task (e.g., Do [\\\/] and [\\\/] match?) taps visuospatial processing but makes no orthographic demands.
2. The letter case judgment task (e.g., Do [bbBb] and [bbBb] match in the pattern of upper- and lowercase letters?) adds an orthographic processing demand but makes no phonological demands because the stimulus items, which consist entirely of consonant strings, are therefore phonotactically impermissible.
3. The single-letter rhyme (e.g., Do the letters [T] and [V] rhyme?) is orthographically more simple than letter case judgment but adds a phonological processing demand, requiring the transcoding of the letters (orthography) into phonological structures and then a phonological analysis of those structures sufficient to determine that they do or do not rhyme.
4. Nonword rhyme (e.g., Do [leat] and [jete] rhyme?) requires analysis of more complex structures.
5. Semantic category judgment (e.g., Are [corn] and [rice] in the same category?) also makes substantial demands on transcoding from print to phonology (Lukatela and Turvey 1994; Van Orden et al. 1990) but also requires that the printed stimulus items activate particular word representations in the reader's lexicon to arrive at the word's meaning.

A common baseline subtraction condition is used in analysis: letter case, single-letter rhyme, nonword rhyme, and semantic category tasks contrasted with the nonlanguage line orientation judgment baseline condition.

Our initial series of investigations examined nonimpaired readers, 19 neurologically normal right-handed men, and 19 women. Figure 3–1 illustrates activations in three subtraction conditions (representing orthographic, phonological, and semantic processing) in two regions of interest (inferior frontal gyrus and extrastriate). In the inferior frontal gyrus, activations during phonological processing were significantly greater than activations during either orthographic or semantic processing. These findings are consonant with those of previous functional imaging studies that show

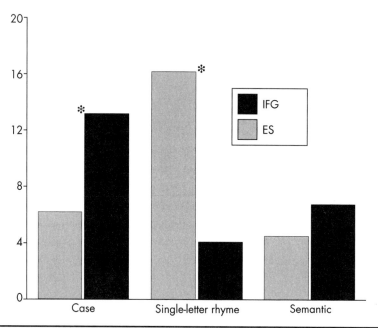

Figure 3–1.   Ordinate represents mean activations for letter case judgment, single-letter rhyme, and semantic category judgment subtractions in the inferior frontal gyrus (IFG) and extrastriate (ES) regions, respectively. In the IFG region, rhyme significantly differed from both case and semantic. In the ES region, case significantly differed from both rhyme and semantic. * = statistically significant difference.

activation in this region in speech production tasks (Petersen et al. 1989), in complex discriminations of speech tokens (Demonet et al. 1992, 1994; Zatorre et al. 1992), in phonological judgments on visually presented single-letter displays (Sergent et al. 1992), and in word/nonword discriminations on visual stimuli (Price et al. 1993). Our findings also are consonant with those of studies of patients with lesions in this region who show evidence of problems with phonetic discriminations (Blumstein et al. 1977). In contrast, in extrastriate regions, activations during orthographic subtractions were significantly greater than activations during either phonological or semantic processing. This finding, that orthographic processing makes maximum demands on extrastriate sites, is consistent with claims made by Petersen and colleagues (Petersen and Fiez 1993; Petersen et al. 1989) after using different tasks in several PET studies. Activations during phonological processing also were observed at sites in both the superior temporal gyrus and the middle temporal gyrus, areas that fall within traditional language regions. However, semantic processing activated both of these areas significantly more strongly than did phonological processing, suggesting that these regions subserved both phonological and lexical semantic processing. The most natural conclusion is that the temporal sites examined are multifunctional, relevant for both phonological and lexical semantic processing, an interpretation supported by previous PET studies (Demonet et al. 1992; Petersen et al. 1989; R. Wise et al. 1991) and our previous fMRI study (B. A. Shaywitz et al. 1995b). Furthermore, lesion studies have suggested that damage to temporal and temporoparietal sites results in semantic deficits (Hart and Gordon 1990).

In this study, we also observed differences in brain activation during phonological processing between men and women. This is illustrated in Figure 3–2, which shows activations during phonological processing for each hemisphere and sex. For comparison, two regions of interest are shown. In the extrastriate region, no significant hemisphere differences in activations are seen for either men or women. In contrast, in the inferior frontal gyrus, activations are similar for right and left hemispheres in women, but phonological processing results in significantly more activation in the left hemisphere in men. This pattern of activation is further illustrated in Figure 3–3, which shows that activation during phonological processing in men was more lateralized to the left inferior frontal gyrus; in contrast, activation during this same task in women resulted in a more bilateral pattern of activation of this region. These findings provided the first clear evidence of sex differences in the functional organization of the brain for language and indicated that these differences exist primarily at the level of phonological processing. At one level, they support and extend a long-held hypothesis that suggested that language functions are more likely to be highly lateralized in men but represented in both cerebral hemispheres in women (Halpern 1992; Witelson and Kigar 1992). Because of this initial finding of sex differences in functional activation within the inferior frontal gyrus, we have obtained three replications of the same basic sex by hemisphere

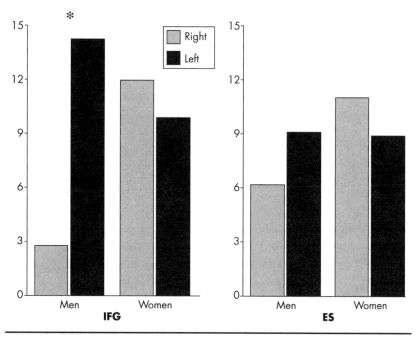

Figure 3–2. Ordinate represents mean activations for men and women, across tasks, in the inferior frontal gyrus (IFG) and extrastriate (ES) regions. In the ES region, no significant hemisphere differences in activations are seen for either men or women. In contrast, in the IFG, activations are similar for right and left hemispheres in women, but phonological processing results in significantly more activation in the left hemisphere in men. * = statistically significant difference.

pattern. In summary, the evidence from several imaging experiments seems clear—the modal pattern at the inferior frontal gyrus indicates relatively greater right-hemisphere involvement for women than for men at the inferior frontal gyrus.

As reviewed earlier in this chapter, previous efforts using functional imaging methods to examine brain organization in dyslexia have been inconclusive (Eden et al. 1996; Flowers et al. 1991; Gross-Glenn et al. 1991; Paulesu et al. 1996; Rumsey et al. 1992, 1997; Salmelin et al. 1996) largely, we think, because the experimental tasks tapped several aspects of the reading process in somewhat unsystematic ways. Our aim, therefore, was to develop a set of hierarchically structured tasks that control the kind of language-

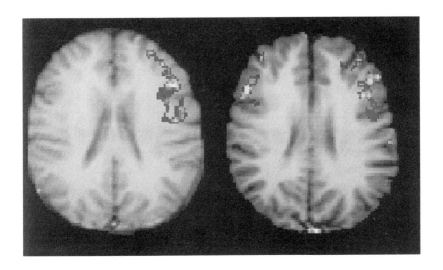

Figure 3–3. Composite brain activations in 19 men (left) and 19 women (right). During rhyming, men activated the left inferior frontal gyrus. In contrast, women activated both left and right inferior frontal gyrus during the same task. Both men and women performed the task equally accurately.

relevant coding required, including especially the demand on phonological analysis, and then to compare the performance and brain activation patterns (as measured by fMRI) of dyslexic and nonimpaired readers. Thus, proceeding from the base of the hierarchy to the top, the tasks made demands on visuospatial processing, orthographic processing, simple phonological analysis, complex phonological analysis, and lexical semantic judgment. We hypothesized that differences in brain activation patterns would emerge as dyslexic and nonimpaired readers were asked to perform tasks that made progressively greater demands on phonological analysis. These tasks, which were described earlier in this chapter, are shown in Table 3–1.

We studied 29 dyslexic and 32 nonimpaired men and women, all in the average range for IQ. Reading performance in the dyslexic subjects was significantly impaired: the mean standard score on a measure of nonword reading was 81 in dyslexic and 114 in nonimpaired readers, with no overlap between groups. Error patterns on the fMRI tasks revealed that dyslexic differed from nonimpaired readers most strikingly on the nonword rhyme task. Nonword reading is perhaps the clearest indication of decoding ability because familiarity with the letter pattern cannot influence the individual's response.

We focused on brain regions of interest that previous research had implicated in reading and language (Demonet et al. 1994; Henderson 1986; Petersen et al. 1990; Pugh et al. 1996) and examined these for evidence of differences between the two reading groups in patterns of activation across the series of tasks. Previous investigators have assumed the existence of a posterior cortical system adapted for reading, a system including Wernicke's area, the angular gyrus, the extrastriate cortex, and the striate cortex (Benson 1994; Black and Behrmann 1994; Geschwind 1965). As shown in Figure 3–4 (top panels) and Figure 3–5, we found differences between dyslexic and nonimpaired readers in the patterns of activation in several critical components of this system: posterior superior temporal gyrus (Wernicke's area), BA 39 (angular gyrus), and BA 17 (striate cortex). The pattern of group differences was similar at each of these sites: nonimpaired readers showed a systematic increase in activation in going from letter case judgment to single-letter rhyme to nonword rhyme (i.e., as orthographic to phonological coding demands increased), whereas dyslexic readers failed to show such systematic modulation in their activation patterns in response to the same task demands. In addition, an anterior region, inferior frontal gyrus, showed significant differences in the pattern of activation between nonimpaired and dyslexic readers (Figure 3–4, bottom panel, and Figure 3–5). However, here, in contrast to findings in the posterior system, dyslexic readers had greater activation than nonimpaired readers in response to increasing phonological decoding demands.

Hemispheric differences between nonimpaired and dyslexic readers have long been suspected (Galaburda et al. 1985; Geschwind 1985; Rumsey et al. 1992; Salmelin et al. 1996) and were found in two regions: the angular gyrus and the parietotemporo-occipital region. In each case, activations in these regions in nonimpaired readers were greater in the left hemisphere, and in contrast, activations in these regions in dyslexic readers were greater in the right hemisphere. This pattern was observed across all tasks. Based on our earlier work (B. A. Shaywitz et al. 1995c), we examined for hemispheric differences between men and women. In the inferior frontal gyrus, a significant sex difference was found: during nonword rhyme, men showed significantly greater activation in the left hemisphere than in the right hemisphere, whereas women showed relatively greater right-hemisphere activation than did men, which is consistent with previous observations.

In this study, we found significant differences in brain activation patterns between dyslexic and nonimpaired readers, differences that emerged during tasks that made progressive demands on phonological analysis. These findings relate the cognitive-behavioral deficit characterizing dyslexic readers to anomalous activation patterns in both posterior and anterior brain regions (Figure 3–5). Thus, within a large posterior cortical system, including Wernicke's area, the angular gyrus, the extrastriate, and the striate cortex, dyslexic readers failed to systematically increase activation as the difficulty of mapping print onto phonological structures increased. In contrast, in anterior regions, including the inferior frontal gyrus and prefrontal regions, dyslexic readers showed a pattern of overactivation in response to even the simplest phonological task (single-letter rhyme) (Figure 3–4). For nonimpaired readers, these data provide functional evidence of a widely distributed computational system for reading characterized by specialization and reciprocity: within the system, task-specific responses vary from region to region. For example, in the inferior frontal gyrus, only the complex phonological task (nonword rhyme) produced a significant increase in activation relative to the orthographic (case judgment) task, suggesting that this region is engaged in letter to sound transcoding; in Wernicke's area, both simple (single-letter rhyme) and more complex (nonword rhyme) phonological tasks produced significant increases in activation relative to the orthographic task, implying that this region processes information in a more abstract phonological form.

What is particularly interesting is that the findings from this most recent functional imaging study of dyslexia now help reconcile the seemingly contradictory findings of previous imaging

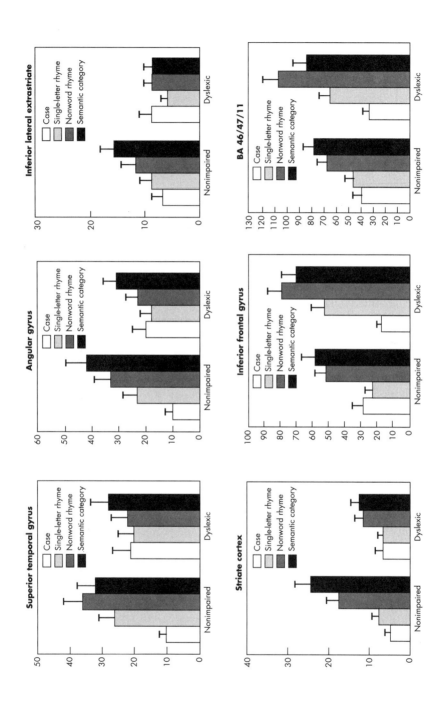

Figure 3-4. Mean number of activated pixels for brain regions where activation patterns across tasks differed significantly between nonimpaired and dyslexic readers. Mean activations ± SEM are shown on ordinate; tasks are shown on abscissa. We found differences between dyslexic and nonimpaired readers in the patterns of activation in several critical components of this system: posterior superior temporal gyrus (Wernicke's area), Brodmann area (BA) 39 (angular gyrus), and BA 17 (striate cortex). The pattern of group differences was similar at each of these sites: nonimpaired subjects showed a systematic increase in activation in going from letter case judgment to single-letter rhyme to nonword rhyme (i.e., as orthographic to phonological coding demands increase), whereas dyslexic readers failed to show such systematic modulation in their activation patterns in response to the same task demands. In addition, an anterior region, inferior frontal gyrus, showed significant differences in the pattern of activation between nonimpaired and dyslexic readers. However, here, in contrast to findings in the posterior system, dyslexic readers had greater activation than nonimpaired readers in response to increasing phonological decoding demands.

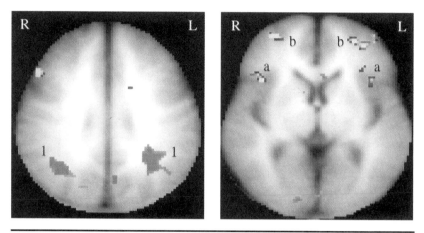

Figure 3–5. Composite activation maps in dyslexic (right panel) and nonimpaired (left panel) readers during phonological processing. During phonological processing, dyslexic readers showed more activation than nonimpaired readers anteriorly in the inferior frontal gyrus bilaterally (a) and in the middle frontal gyrus (b). In contrast, nonimpaired readers activated a large area in the posterior region, the angular gyrus (1).

studies of dyslexia, some of which involved anomalous findings in the visual system (Demb 1998; Eden et al. 1996), but others indicated abnormal activation within components of the language system (Flowers et al. 1991; Gross-Glenn et al. 1991; Paulesu et al. 1996; Rumsey et al. 1992, 1997; Salmelin et al. 1996). These data indicate that dyslexic readers have a functional disruption in an extensive system in the posterior cortex, encompassing both traditional visual and traditional language regions as well as a portion of association cortex. The involvement of this latter region centered about the angular gyrus is of particular interest because this portion of association cortex is considered pivotal in carrying out those cross-modal integrations necessary for reading (i.e., mapping the visual percept of the print onto the phonological structures of the language [Benson 1994; Black and Behrmann 1994; Geschwind 1965]). Consistent with this study of developmental dyslexia, a large literature on acquired inability to read (alexia) describes neuroanatomical lesions most prominently centered about the angular gyrus (Damasio 1983; Dejerine 1891; Friedman et al. 1993). It should not be surprising that both the acquired and the developmental disorders affecting reading have in common a disruption within the neural systems serving to link the visual representations of the letters to the phonological structures they represent. Although reading difficulty is the primary symptom in both acquired alexia and developmental dyslexia, associated symptoms and findings in the two disorders would be expected to differ somewhat, reflecting the differences between an acquired and a developmental disorder. In acquired alexia, a structural lesion resulting from an insult (e.g., stroke, tumor) disrupts a component of an already functioning neural system, and the lesion may extend to involve other brain regions and systems. In developmental dyslexia, as a result of a constitutionally based functional disruption, the system never develops normally so that the symptoms reflect the emanative effects of an early disruption to the phonological system. In either case, the disruption is within the same neuroanatomical system.

For dyslexic readers, these brain activation patterns provide evidence of an imperfectly functioning system for segmenting words into their phonological constituents; accordingly, this disruption is evident when dyslexic readers are asked to respond to increasing demands on phonological analysis. These findings add neurobiological support for previous cognitive-behavioral data pointing to the critical role of phonological analysis, and its impairment, in dyslexia. The pattern of relative underactivation in posterior brain regions contrasted with relative overactivation in anterior regions may provide a neural signature for the phonological difficulties characterizing dyslexia.

Diagnosis and Evaluation of Dyslexia

The advances in the understanding of the cognitive and neurobiological basis of dyslexia significantly influence how we diagnose and, ultimately, how we most effectively treat dyslexia in children and young adults. Guided by this knowledge of the presumed underlying pathophysiology, the clinician seeks to determine through history, observation, and psychometric assessment 1) whether the patient has difficulties in reading that are unexpected, given the person's age, intelligence, or level of education, and 2) whether the patient has associated linguistic problems at the level of phonological processing. How reading and language are assessed depends on the age and educational level of the patient. As in most diagnoses in medicine, the history is critical. Clues to the diagnosis of dyslexia in the school-age child include a history of delayed language; problems with the sounds of words, such as trouble rhyming words and difficulty learning to associate the sounds with the letters; and, of particular importance, a history of reading and spelling difficulties in the parents and siblings. Current reading performance in school provides additional clues: difficulty decoding single words, the difficulty most apparent when decoding nonsense words or unfamiliar words; slow reading; comprehension often superior to isolated decoding skills; and problems in spelling. Reading ability is assessed by the measurement of decoding skills and comprehension. In the school-age child, the most important element of the psychometric evaluation is how accurately the child can decode words—that is, read single words in isolation. Reading passages allows bright children with dyslexia to use the context to guess the meaning of a word they might otherwise have trouble decoding. As a result, readers with dyslexia often perform better on measures of comprehension and worse on measures of the ability to decode isolated single words. In practice, the reliance on context makes tests such as multiple-choice examinations, which typically provide scanty context, especially burdensome for readers with dyslexia. Residents often ask us whether they, as practicing physicians, should test the children themselves. In our experience, it is far more reasonable for physicians to know how to interpret the reading measures than to administer them.

The role of intelligence tests in the diagnosis of dyslexia is controversial (Fletcher et al. 1996; Shankweiler et al. 1995). Traditionally, the concept of dyslexia as an unexpected difficulty in reading has been interpreted as underachievement in reading relative to ability (IQ)—that is, a discrepancy between the level of reading achievement predicted on the basis of IQ and the actual level of reading achievement. Consequently, IQ tests are generally used to assess dyslexia in school-age children, and, in fact, eligibility for special education programs in public schools usually is based on the identification of an ability–achievement discrepancy. More recently, many have questioned the requirement of such a discrepancy (Bruck 1992; Stanovich and Siegel 1994). The issue is complex. In certain respects, children with dyslexia identified on the basis of an ability–achievement discrepancy do not seem different from those of average intelligence whose dyslexia is identified solely on the basis of low reading achievement for chronological age; both have a deficit in phonological processing (Bruck 1992; Stanovich and Siegel 1994) and follow the same developmental trajectory in reading. At the same time, it should be recognized that the use of an approach based on such a discrepancy in the diagnosis of dyslexia is important for the identification of very bright children who have dyslexia.

Approximately 75% of the children whose dyslexia meets the criteria for a discrepancy between ability and achievement also have low reading achievement (S. E. Shaywitz et al. 1992); however, the remaining 25% of the children meeting discrepancy criteria—most of whom are extremely bright and also manifest a phonological deficit—do not meet low-achievement criteria and would be excluded from special education services if the low-achievement criterion were the only one used. Thus, a consensus is developing that in school-age children, the criterion of "unexpected" reading difficulties may be met by children of at least average intelligence who meet either discrepancy criteria relative to IQ or low-achievement criteria relative to chronological age (Brown et al. 1993; S. E. Shaywitz 1996).

Currently, most children's reading disability is not diagnosed until they are in third grade, or about 9 years old (Lyon et al. 1997). The application of what has been learned about the acquisition of reading and the availability of tests of phonological skills now make it possible, first, to identify children with dyslexia even before they fail in reading (Torgesen 1995) and, second, to provide appropriate early interventions. A history of language delay or of not attending to the sounds of words (trouble playing rhyming games with words or confusing words that sound alike), along with a family history, are important risk factors for dyslexia. The most helpful measures in predicting difficulties are phonemic awareness and letter knowledge.

Special Considerations: Diagnosis and Evaluation of Dyslexia in Young Adults

Given the considerable number of psychiatrists who see adolescence and adults, we emphasize the implications of what we have learned about dyslexia on the diagnosis and management of dyslexia in a frequently overlooked group of individuals—bright young adults. The developmental course of dyslexia now has been characterized. First, dyslexia is persistent; it does not go away (Francis et al. 1996; Shaywitz et al. 1995a). On a practical level, this means that once a person is given a diagnosis of dyslexia, reexamination after high school to confirm the diagnosis is unnecessary. Second, over the course of development, the ability to decode words becomes more accurate and automatic in skilled readers; they do not need to rely on context for word identification. Readers with dyslexia, too, become more accurate over time, but they do not become automatic. Residua of the phonological deficit persist (Bruck 1992; Felton et al. 1990) so that reading remains effortful, even for the brightest people with childhood histories of dyslexia (Lefly and Pennington 1991). The failure either to recognize or to measure the lack of automaticity in reading is, perhaps, the most common error in the diagnosis of dyslexia in accomplished young adults. It is often not understood that tests measuring word accuracy may be inadequate for the diagnosis of dyslexia in young adults at the level of college or graduate or professional school and that for these people, timed measures of reading must be used to make the diagnosis. However, very few standardized tests for adult readers are administered under timed and untimed conditions; the Nelson-Denny Reading Test (Brown et al. 1993) is an exception. The reading measures (Woodcock and Johnson 1989) commonly used for school-age children may provide misleading data on some adolescents and young adults because they assess reading accuracy but not automaticity (speed).

For bright young adults especially, the history is perhaps the most sensitive and accurate indicator of dyslexia. A history of phonologically based language difficulties (e.g., mispronouncing words, speech punctuated by hesitations and dysfluencies), of trouble reading new or unfamiliar words, of spelling difficulties,

Table 3–2. Clues to dyslexia in school-age children

History

Delayed language

Problems with the sounds of words (trouble rhyming words, confusion of words that sound alike)

Expressive language difficulties (mispronunciations, hesitations, word-finding difficulties)

Difficulty naming (difficulty learning the letters of the alphabet and the names of numbers)

Difficulty learning to associate sounds with letters

History of reading and spelling difficulties in parents and siblings

Reading

Difficulty decoding single words

Particular difficulty reading nonsense or unfamiliar words

Inaccurate and labored oral reading

Slow reading

Comprehension often superior to isolated decoding skills

Poor spelling

Language

Relatively poor performance on tests of word retrieval (name the pictured item)

Relatively superior performance on tests of word recognition (point to the pictured item)

Poor performance on tests of phonological awareness

and of requiring additional time for reading and taking tests relative to the level of education achieved represents the distinct diagnostic signature of dyslexia.

Tests of reading, spelling, language, and cognitive abilities (for school-age children) represent a core battery for the diagnosis of dyslexia; additional tests of academic achievement (in mathematics, for example) or memory may be administered as part of a more comprehensive evaluation of academic, linguistic, or cognitive function. No single test score is pathognomonic of dyslexia. As with any other medical diagnosis, the diagnosis of dyslexia should reflect a thoughtful synthesis of all the clinical data available, including the history, observations, and testing data (Table 3–2). The clinician is seeking converging evidence of a phonologically based reading disability, as indicated by a disparity between the person's reading and phonological skills and his or her intellectual capabilities, age, or level of education. Dyslexia is distinguished from other disorders that may feature reading difficulties prominently by the unique, circumscribed nature of the phonological deficit, one that does not intrude into other linguistic or cognitive domains (Table 3–3). Primary sensory impairments should be ruled out, particularly in young children; other laboratory measures, such as imaging studies, electroencephalography, or genetic tests, are ordered only if there are specific clinical indications. Although there have been important advances in the use of imaging to study cognitive function, such technology is still reserved for investigational purposes.

Attention-deficit/hyperactivity disorder also may affect learning in both children and adults. It is an entirely different disorder from dyslexia; they differ in their proposed mechanisms, symptoms, assessments, and interventions (B. A. Shaywitz et al. 1995). A proportion of patients with dyslexia (12%–24%) (S. E. Shaywitz et al. 1994) also will have attention-deficit/hyperactivity disorder, and if there is any suggestion that inattention may be a problem, the patient should be examined for specific symptoms that meet the DSM-IV (American Psychiatric Association 1994) criteria for attention-deficit/hyperactivity disorder.

Management of Dyslexia

The management of dyslexia demands a life-span perspective; early on, the focus is on remediation. As a child matures and enters the more time-demanding setting of secondary school, the emphasis shifts to the important role of providing accommodations. Because physicians are frequently asked about various reading programs for dyslexia, they should understand the key elements of an effective training program.

To learn to read, all children must discover that spoken words can be broken down into smaller units of sound, that letters on the page represent these sounds, and that written words have the same number and sequence of sounds heard in the spoken word.

Table 3–3. Some disorders that may present with reading difficulties

Developmental dyslexia

Phonological deficit primary

Reading impairment at the level of single-word decoding

Other components of language system intact (e.g., syntax, semantics)

Intelligence not affected and may be in superior or gifted range

Language-learning disability[a]

Primary deficit involves all aspects of language, both phonological and
  semantic syntactic

Reading difficulty at the level of both decoding and comprehension

Prominent language difficulties

Measures of verbal intelligence significantly affected by language
  deficit; may be in subaverage range

Acquired alexia[b]

Loss or diminution of reading ability

Result of trauma, tumor, or stroke (e.g., occlusion of posterior cerebral
  artery)

Several forms reflecting specific loci of neuroanatomical lesions (e.g.,
  alexia with or without agraphia)

May be accompanied by other features reflecting locus and extent of the
  lesion

Hyperlexia[c]

Word-recognition ability substantially better than reading
  comprehension

Early intense interest in words and letters

Exceptional word-recognition ability, apparent by age 5 years

Very poor reading comprehension

Disordered language development, especially affecting aural
  comprehension

Deficits in reasoning and abstract problem-solving

Behavioral atypicalities affecting interpersonal relationships

---

[a]Discussed in Catts and Kamhi (in press).
[b]Discussed in Damasio and Damasio (1983).
[c]Discussed in Aram and Healy (1988).

When children have made these associations, usually by the end
of first grade, they have discovered the *alphabetic principle* and
have essentially broken the reading code. Children with dyslexia

do not easily acquire the basic phonological skills that are a prerequisite to reading; consequently, concepts such as phoneme awareness must be taught explicitly. Operationally, this is accomplished with systematic and highly structured training exercises, such as identifying rhyming and nonrhyming word pairs, blending isolated sounds to form a word, or conversely, segmenting a spoken word into its individual sounds. Furthermore, it is now recognized that awareness of phonemes is necessary but not sufficient for learning to read (Gough and Tunmer 1986). In addition to learning that words can be segmented into smaller units of sound (phoneme awareness) and that these sounds are linked to specific letters and letter patterns (phonics), children with dyslexia require practice in reading stories, both to allow them to apply their newly acquired decoding skills to reading words in context and to experience reading for meaning (Lyon et al. 1997).

Several protocols differing in method, format, intensity, and duration of the reading intervention are being tested in large-scale studies; data from these trials should provide important information to clarify further which specific programs are most effective for particular groups of children with dyslexia (Lyon and Moats 1997). Large-scale studies to date have focused on younger children; as yet, few or no data are available on the effect of these training programs on older children. People with dyslexia and their families frequently consult their physicians about unconventional approaches to the remediation of reading difficulties; in general, very few credible data support the claims made for these treatments (e.g., optometric training, medication for vestibular dysfunction, chiropractic manipulation, and dietary supplementation) (Silver 1995).

The management of dyslexia in students in secondary school, and especially college and graduate school, is based on accommodation rather than remediation. College students with a history of childhood dyslexia often present a paradoxical picture; they are similar to their nonimpaired peers on measures of word recognition yet continue to have the phonological deficit that makes reading less automatic, more effortful, and slow (Bruck 1992; Felton et al. 1990). For these readers with dyslexia, the provision of extra time is an essential accommodation; this time allows them to decode each word and to apply their unimpaired higher-order cognitive and linguistic skills to the surrounding context to grasp the meaning of words that they cannot entirely or rapidly decode. Although providing extra time for reading is by far the most common accommodation for people with dyslexia, other helpful accommodations include allowing the use of laptop computers with spelling checkers, tape recorders in the classroom, and recorded books (materials are available from Recording for the Blind and Dyslexic, 800-221-4792) and providing access to syllabi and lecture notes, tutors to "talk through" and review the content of reading material, alternatives to multiple-choice tests (e.g., reports or orally administered tests), and a separate, quiet room for taking tests. With such accommodations, many students with dyslexia are now successfully completing studies in a range of disciplines, including medicine.

Conclusions and Implications

Within the last two decades, overwhelming evidence from many laboratories has converged to indicate the cognitive basis for dyslexia: dyslexia represents a disorder within the language system and, more specifically, within a particular subcomponent of that system—phonological processing. Recent advances in imaging technology and the development of tasks that sharply isolate the subcomponent processes of reading now allow phonological processing to be localized in the brain and, as a result, provide for the first time the potential for elucidating a biological signature for reading and reading disability.

The discovery of a neuroanatomical locus unique to phonological processing has significant implications. At the most fundamental level, it is now possible to investigate specific hypotheses regarding the neural substrate of dyslexia and to verify, reject, or modify suggested cognitive models. From a more clinical perspective, the isolation of phonological processing in the brain and, with it, a potential biological signature for dyslexia offers the promise for more precise identification and diagnosis of dyslexia and ultimately a more successful treatment of this most common disorder in children, adolescents, and adults.

The isolated nature of the phonological deficit in dyslexia has important clinical implications. It means that other higher-order cognitive functions such as vocabulary, reasoning, and conceptualization and analytic abilities are not only intact but also often highly developed. Many leaders in medicine and science, including Loretta Bender, Carl Jung, Harvey Cushing, Helen Taussig, Ron David, and Nobel Laureates Barry Benacerref and Niels Bohr, have been dyslexic.

References

Anderson A, Gore J: The physical basis of neuroimaging techniques, in Child and Adolescent Psychiatric Clinics of North America, Vol 6. Edited by Lewis M, Peterson B. Philadelphia, PA, WB Saunders, 1997, pp 213–264

American Psychiatric Association: Diagnostic and Statistical Manual of Mental Disorders, 4th Edition. Washington, DC, American Psychiatric Association, 1994

Aram, D, Healy J: Hyperlexia: a review of extraordinary word recognition, in The Exceptional Brain: Neuropsychology of Talent and Special Abilities. Edited by Obler L, Fein D. New York, Guilford, 1988, pp 70–102

Ball EW, Blachman BA: Does phoneme awareness training in kindergarten make a difference in early word recognition and developmental spelling? Reading Research Quarterly 26(1):49–66, 1991

Benson DF: The Neurology of Thinking. New York, Oxford University Press, 1994

Black SE, Behrmann M: Localization in alexia, in Localization and Neuroimaging in Neuropsychology. Edited by Kertesz A. New York, Academic Press, 1994, pp 331–376

Bloomfield L: Language. New York, Spansuls, Rinehart & Winston, 1933

Blumstein SE, Baker E, Goodglass H: Phonological factors in auditory comprehension in aphasia. Neuropsychologia 15:19–30, 1977

Bradley L, Bryant PE: Categorizing sounds and learning to read—a causal connection. Nature 301:419–421, 1983

Brady SA, Shankweiler DP (eds): Phonological Processes in Literacy: A Tribute to Isabelle Y. Liberman. Hillsdale, NJ, Lawrence Erlbaum, 1991

Brown JI, Fishco VV, Hanna GS: Nelson-Denny Reading Test, Forms G and H. Itasca, IL, Riverside Publishing, 1993

Bruck M: Persistence of dyslexics' phonological awareness deficits. Dev Psychol 28:874–886, 1992

Catts H, Kamhi A: Defining reading disabilities, in Language Basis of Reading Disabilities. Edited by Catts H, Kamhi A (eds). Boston, MA, Allyn & Bacon (in press)

Damasio AR: Pure alexia. Trends Neurosci 6(3):93–96, 1983

Damasio A, Damasio H: The anatomic basis of pure alexia. Neurology 33:1573–1583, 1983

Damasio AR, Damasio H: Brain and language. Sci Am 267:89–95, 1992

Dejerine J: Sur un cas de cécité verbale avec agraphie, suivi d'autopsie. C R Société du Biologie 43:197–201, 1891

Demb J, Boynton G, Heeger D: Functional magnetic resonance imaging of early visual pathways in dyslexia. J Neurosci 18:6939–6951, 1998

Demonet JF, Chollet F, Ramsey S, et al: The anatomy of phonological and semantic processing in normal subjects. Brain 115:1753–1768, 1992

Demonet JF, Price C, Wise R, et al: A PET study of cognitive strategies in normal subjects during language tasks: influence of phonetic ambiguity and sequence processing on phoneme monitoring. Brain 117:671–682, 1994

Denckla MB, LeMay M, Chapman CA: Few CT scan abnormalities found even in neurologically impaired learning disabled children. J Learn Disabil 18:132–135, 1985

Dool CB, Steimack RM, Rourke BP: Event-related potentials in children with learning disabilities. J Clin Child Psychol 22:387–398, 1993

Duara R, Kushch A, Gross-Glenn K, et al: Neuroanatomic differences between dyslexic and normal readers on magnetic resonance imaging scans. Arch Neurol 48:410–416, 1991

Eden GF, Stein JF, Wood HM, et al: Differences in visuospatial judgement in reading-disabled and normal children. Percept Mot Skills 82:155–177, 1996

Felton RH, Naylor CE, Wood FB: Neuropsychological profile of adult dyslexics. Brain Lang 39:485–497, 1990

Finucci JM, Childs B: Are there really more dyslexic boys than girls? in Sex Differences in Dyslexia. Edited by Ansara A, Geschwind N, Albert M, et al. Towson, MD, Orton Dyslexia Society, 1981, pp 1–9

Fletcher JM, Shaywitz SE, Shankweiler DP, et al: Cognitive profiles of reading disability: comparisons of discrepancy and low achievement definitions. J Educ Psychol 86(1):6–23, 1994

Fletcher JM, Francis DJ, Stuebing KK, et al: Conceptual and methodological issues in construct definition, in Attention, Memory, and Executive Function. Edited by Lyon GR, Krasnegor NA. Baltimore, MD, Paul H. Brookes, 1996, pp 17–42

Flowers DL, Wood FB, Naylor CE: Regional cerebral blood flow correlates of language processes in reading disability. Arch Neurol 48:637–643, 1991

Flynn JM, Rahbar MH: Prevalence of reading failure in boys compared with girls. Psychology in the Schools 31:66–71, 1994

Foorman BR, Francis DJ, Beeler T, et al: Early interventions for children with reading problems: study designs and preliminary findings. Learning Disabilities: A Multidisciplinary Journal 8(1):63–71, 1997

Francis DJ, Shaywitz SE, Stuebing KK, et al: Developmental lag versus deficit models of reading disability: a longitudinal, individual growth curves analysis. J Educ Psychol 88(1):3–17, 1996

Friedman RF, Ween JE, Albert ML: Alexia, in Clinical Neuropsychology, 3rd Edition. Edited by Heilman KM, Valenstein E. New York, Oxford University Press, 1993, pp 37–62

Friston KJ, Frith CD, Liddle PF, et al: Functional connectivity: the principal-component analysis of large (PET) data sets. Journal of Cerebral Blood Flow and Metabolism 13:5–14, 1993

Galaburda AM, Kemper TL: Cytoarchitectonic abnormalities in developmental dyslexia: a case study. Ann Neurol 6:94–100, 1979

Galaburda AM, Sherman GF, Rosen GD, et al: Developmental dyslexia: four consecutive patients with cortical anomalies. Ann Neurol 18:222–233, 1985

Geschwind N: Disconnection syndromes in animals and man. Brain 88:237–294, 1965

Geschwind N: Biological foundations of reading, in Dyslexia: A Neuroscientific Approach to Clinical Evaluation. Edited by Duffy FH, Geschwind N. Boston, MA, Little, Brown, 1985, pp 195–211

Gilger JW, Borecki IB, Smith SD, et al: The etiology of extreme scores for complex phenotypes: an illustration using reading performance, in Developmental Dyslexia: Neural, Cognitive, and Genetic Mechanisms. Edited by Chase CH, Rosen GD, Sherman GF. Baltimore, MD, York Press, 1996, pp 63–85

Gough PB, Tunmer WE: Decoding, reading, and reading disability. Remedial and Special Education 7:6–10, 1986

Gross-Glenn K, Duara R, Barker WW, et al: Positron emission tomographic studies during serial word-reading by normal and dyslexic adults. J Clin Exp Neuropsychol 13:531–544, 1991

Halpern DF: Sex Differences in Cognitive Abilities, 2nd Edition. Hillsdale, NJ, Lawrence Erlbaum, 1992

Hart J, Gordon B: Delineation of single-word semantic comprehension deficits in aphasia, with anatomical correlation. Ann Neurol 27:226–231, 1990

Haslam RHA, Dalby JT, Johns RD, et al: Cerebral asymmetry in developmental dyslexia. Arch Neurol 38:679–682, 1981

Henderson VW: Anatomy of posterior pathways in reading: a reassessment. Brain Lang 29:119–133, 1986

Hier DB, LeMay M, Rosenberger PB, et al: Developmental dyslexia: evidence for a subgroup with a reversal of cerebral asymmetry. Arch Neurol 35:90–92, 1978

Hughes JR: Electroencephalographic and neurophysiological studies in dyslexia, in Dyslexia: An Appraisal of Current Knowledge. Edited by Benton AL, Pearl D. New York, Oxford University Press, 1977, pp 205–240

Humphreys P, Kaufmann WE, Galaburda AM: Developmental dyslexia in women: neuropathological findings in three patients. Ann Neurol 28:727–738, 1990

Hynd GW, Semrud-Clikeman M: Dyslexia and brain morphology. Psychol Bull 106:447–482, 1989

Hynd GW, Semrud-Clikeman M, Lorys AR, et al: Brain morphology in developmental dyslexia and attention deficit disorder/hyperactivity. Arch Neurol 47:919–926, 1990

Interagency Committee on Learning Disabilities: Learning Disabilities: A Report to the U.S. Congress. Washington, DC, U.S. Government Printing Office, 1987

Jernigan TL, Hesselink JR, Sowell E, et al: Cerebral structure on magnetic resonance imaging in language- and learning-impaired children. Arch Neurol 48:539–545, 1991

Larsen JP, Høien T, Lundberg I, et al: MRI evaluation of the size and symmetry of the planum temporale in adolescents with developmental dyslexia. Brain Lang 39:289–301, 1990

Lefly DL, Pennington BF: Spelling errors and reading fluency in compensated adult dyslexics. Annals of Dyslexia 41:143–162, 1991

Leisman G, Ashkenazi M: Aetiological factors in dyslexia, IV: cerebral hemispheres are functionally equivalent. Neurosci Biobehav Rev 11:157–164, 1980

LeMay M: Are there radiological changes in the brains of individuals with dyslexia? Bulletin of the Orton Society 31:135–141, 1981

Leonard CM, Voeller KS, Lombardino LJ, et al: Anomalous cerebral structure in dyslexia revealed with magnetic resonance imaging. Arch Neurol 50:461–469, 1993

Lerner JW: Educational interventions in learning disabilities. J Am Acad Child Adolesc Psychiatry 28:326–331, 1989

Liberman AM: Speech: A Special Code. Cambridge, MA, MIT Press, 1996

Liberman AM: When theories of speech meet the real world. J Psycholinguist Res 27:111–122, 1998

Liberman IY, Shankweiler D, Liberman AM: Phonology and reading disability: solving the reading puzzle, in International Academy for Research in Learning Disabilities Monograph Series, Vol 6. Edited by Shankweiler D, Liberman IY. Ann Arbor, University of Michigan Press, 1989, pp 1–33

Lou HC, Henriksen L, Bruhn P: Focal cerebral hypoperfusion in children with dysphasia and/or attention deficit disorder. Arch Neurol 42:825–829, 1984

Lou HC, Henriksen L, Bruhn P: Focal cerebral dysfunction in developmental learning disabilities. Lancet 335:8–11, 1990

Lukatela G, Turvey MT: Visual lexical access is initially phonological, 2: evidence from phonological priming by homophones and pseudohomophones. J Exp Psychol Gen 123:331–353, 1994

Lyon Gr, Moats LC: Critical, conceptual, and methodological considerations in reading intervention research. J Learn Disabil 30:578–588, 1997

Lyon GR, Alexander D, Yaffee S: Progress and promise in research in learning disabilities. Learning Disabilities: A Multidisciplinary Journal 8(1):1–6, 1997

Nicolson RI, Fawcett AJ, Dean P: Time estimation deficits in developmental dyslexia: evidence of cerebellar involvement. Proc R Soc Lond B Biol Sci 259(1354):43–47, 1995

Olson RK, Forsberg H, Wise B: Genes, environment, and the development of orthographic skills, in The Varieties of Orthographic Knowledge, I: Theoretical and Developmental Issues. Edited by Berninger VW. Dordrecht, The Netherlands, Kluwer Academic Publishers, 1994, pp 2–71

Parkins R, Roberts RJ, Reinarz SJ, et al: CT asymmetries in adult developmental dyslexics. Paper presented at the annual convention of the International Neuropsychological Society, Washington, DC, January 1987

Paulesu E, Frith U, Snowling M, et al: Is developmental dyslexia a disconnection syndrome? Evidence from PET scanning. Brain 119:143–157, 1996

Petersen SE, Fiez JA: The processing of single words studied with positron emission tomography. Annu Rev Neurosci 16:509–530, 1993

Petersen SE, Fox PT, Posner MI, et al: Positron emission tomographic studies of the processing of single words. J Cogn Neurosci 1:153–170, 1989

Petersen SE, Fox PT, Snyder AZ, et al: Activation of extrastriate and frontal cortical areas by visual words and word-like stimuli. Science 249:1041–1044, 1990

Pinker S: Rules of language. Science 253:530–535, 1991

Price C, Wise R, Howard D, et al: The brain regions involved in the recognition of visually presented words (abstract). Journal of Cerebral Blood Flow and Metabolism 13:S501, 1993

Pugh KR, Shaywitz BA, Shaywitz SE, et al: Auditory selective attention: an fMRI investigation. Neuroimage 4:159–173, 1996

Rieben L, Perfetti C: Learning to Read: Basic Research and Its Implications. Hillsdale, NJ, Lawrence Erlbaum, 1991

Rosenberger P, Hier D: Cerebral asymmetry and verbal intellectual deficits. Ann Neurol 8:300–304, 1980

Rumsey JM, Dorwart R, Vermess M, et al: Magnetic resonance imaging of brain anatomy in severe developmental dyslexia. Arch Neurol 43:1045–1046, 1986

Rumsey JM, Andreason P, Zametkin AJ, et al: Failure to activate the left temporoparietal cortex in dyslexia. Arch Neurol 49:527–534, 1992

Rumsey JM, Zametkin AJ, Andreason P, et al: Normal activation of frontotemporal language cortex in dyslexia, as measured with oxygen 15 positron emission tomography. Arch Neurol 51:27–38, 1994

Rumsey JM, Nace K, Donohue B, et al: A positron emission tomographic study of impaired word recognition and phonological processing in dyslexic men. Arch Neurol 54:562–573, 1997

Salmelin R, Service E, Kiesila P, et al: Impaired visual word processing in dyslexia revealed with magnetoencephalography. Ann Neurol 40:157–162, 1996

Scarborough HS: Continuity between childhood dyslexia and adult reading. Br J Psychol 75:329–348, 1984

Sergent J: Brain-imaging studies of cognitive function. Trends Neurosci 17:221–227, 1994

Sergent J, Zuck E, Levesque M, et al: Positron emission tomography study of letter and object processing: empirical findings and methodological considerations. Cereb Cortex 2:68–80, 1992

Shankweiler D, Liberman IY, Mark LS, et al: The speech code and learning to read. Journal of Experimental Psychology: Human Learning and Memory 5:531–545, 1979

Shankweiler D, Crain S, Katz L, et al: Cognitive profiles of reading-disabled children: comparison of language skills in phonology, morphology, and syntax. Psychological Science 6(3):149–156, 1995

Shaywitz BA, Holford TR, Holahan JM, et al: A Matthew effect for IQ but not for reading: results from a longitudinal study. Reading Research Quarterly 30(4):894–906, 1995a

Shaywitz BA, Pugh KR, Constable RT, et al: Localization of semantic processing using functional magnetic resonance imaging. Hum Brain Mapp 2:149–158, 1995b

Shaywitz BA, Shaywitz SE, Pugh KR, et al: Sex differences in the functional organization of the brain for language. Nature 373:607–609, 1995c

Shaywitz SE: Dyslexia. Sci Am 275(5):98–104, 1996

Shaywitz SE: Current concepts: dyslexia. N Engl J Med 338:307–312, 1998

Shaywitz SE, Shaywitz BA, Fletcher JM, et al: Prevalence of reading disability in boys and girls: results of the Connecticut Longitudinal Study. JAMA 264:998–1002, 1990

Shaywitz SE, Escobar MD, Shaywitz BA, et al: Evidence that dyslexia may represent the lower tail of a normal distribution of reading ability. N Engl J Med 326:145–150, 1992

Shaywitz SE, Fletcher JM, Shaywitz BA: Issues in the definition and classification of attention deficit disorder. Topics in Language Disorders 14(4):1–25, 1994

Silver LB: Controversial therapies. J Child Neurol 10 (suppl 1):S96–S100, 1995

Stanovich KE, Siegel LS: Phenotypic performance profile of children with reading disabilities: a regression-based test of the phonological-core variable-difference model. J Educ Psychol 86(1):24–53, 1994

Stanovich KE, Cunningham AE, Cramer BB: Assessing phonological awareness in kindergarten children: issues of task comparability. J Exp Child Psychol 38:175–190, 1984

Stein JF: Visuospatial perception in disabled readers, in Visual Processes in Reading and Reading Disabilities. Edited by Willows DM, Kruk RS, Corcos E. Hillsdale, NJ, Lawrence Erlbaum, 1993, pp 331–346

Stein J, Walsh V: To see but not to read; the magnocellular theory of dyslexia. Trends Neurosci 20:147–152, 1997

Swick D, Kutas M, Neville HJ: Localizing the neural genetics of event-related brain potentials, in Localization and Neuroimaging in Neuropsychology. Edited by Kertesz A. New York, Academic Press, 1994, pp 73–121

Tallal P, Stark RE: Perceptual/motor profiles of reading impaired children with or without concomitant oral language deficits. Annals of Dyslexia 32:163–176, 1982

Thatcher RW: Neuroimaging of cyclic cortical reorganization during human development, in Developmental Neuroimaging: Mapping the Development of Brain and Behavior. Edited by Thatcher RW, Lyon GR, Rumsey J, et al. New York, Academic Press, 1996, pp 91–106

Torgesen JK: Phonological Awareness: A Critical Factor in Dyslexia. Baltimore, MD, Orton Dyslexia Society, 1995

Torgesen JK, Morgan ST, Davis C: Effects of two types of phonological awareness training on word learning in kindergarten children. J Educ Psychol 84(3):364–370, 1992

Torgesen JK, Wagner RK, Rashotte CA: Longitudinal studies of phonological processing and reading. J Learn Disabil 27:276–286, 1994

Van Orden GC, Pennington BF, Stone GO: Word identification in reading and the promise of subsymbolic psycholinguistics. Psychol Rev 97:488–522, 1990

Wadsworth SJ, DeFries JC, Stevenson J, et al: Gender ratios among reading-disabled children and their siblings as a function of parental impairment. J Child Psychol Psychiatry 33:1229–1239, 1992

Wise BW, Olson RK: Computer-based phonological awareness and reading instruction. Annals of Dyslexia 45:99–122, 1995

Wise R, Chollet F, Hadar U, et al: Distribution of cortical neural networks involved in word comprehension and word retrieval. Brain 114:1803–1817, 1991

Witelson SF, Kigar DL: Sylvian fissure morphology and asymmetry in men and women: bilateral differences in relation to handedness in men. J Comp Neurol 323:326–340, 1992

Wood F, Flowers L, Buchsbaum M, et al: Investigation of abnormal left temporal functioning in dyslexia through rCBF, auditory evoked potentials, and positron emission tomography. Reading and Writing: An Interdisciplinary Journal 3(379–393):191–205, 1991

Wood FB, Garrett AS, Hart LA, et al: Event related potential correlates of glucose metabolism in normal adults during a cognitive activation task, in Developmental Neuroimaging: Mapping the Development of Brain and Behavior. Edited by Thatcher RW, Lyon GR, Rumsey J, et al. New York, Academic Press, 1996, pp 197–206

Woodcock RW, Johnson MB: Woodcock-Johnson Psycho-Educational Battery—Revised (WJ-R). Allen, TX, Developmental Learning Materials, 1989

Zatorre RJ, Evans AC, Meyer E, et al: Lateralization of phonetic and pitch discrimination in speech processing. Science 256(5058):846–849, 1992

Chapter 4

Evaluation of Learning Disorders in Children With a Psychiatric Disorder

An Example From the Multimodal Treatment Study for ADHD (MTA Study)

James M. Swanson, Ph.D.
Tom Hanley, Ed.D.
Stephen Simpson, M.A.
Mark Davies, M.P.H.
Ann Schulte, Ph.D.
Karen Wells, Ph.D.
Stephen Hinshaw, Ph.D.
Howard Abikoff, Ph.D.
Lily Hechtman, M.D., F.R.C.P.C.
William Pelham, Ph.D.

Betsy Hoza, Ph.D.
Joanne Severe, M.S.
Brooke Molina, Ph.D.
Carol Odbert, B.S.
Steve Forness, Ed.D.
Frank Gresham, Ph.D.
L. Eugene Arnold, M.D., M.Ed.
Timothy Wigal, Ph.D.
Michael Wasdell, M.A.
Laurence L. Greenhill, M.D.

Attention-deficit/hyperactivity disorder (ADHD) and learning disorders (LD) are described in DSM-IV (American Psychiatric Association 1994; pp. 46–63 and 78–85). Similar but not identical conditions (see Arnold 1990) are described in the Individuals With Disabilities Education Act (IDEA) statute, amendments, and regulations, which are reviewed in the 19th Annual Report to Congress (U.S. Department of Education 1998, pp. 36-37). There, the term *disability* (rather than *disorder*) is used, and the category labels are "Other Health Impaired (OHI)" and "Specific Learning Disabilities (SLD)."

By either approach, these are probably separate conditions (Faraone et al. 1993; Felton and Wood 1989) that often co-occur in some individuals (Cantwell and Baker 1992; Shaywitz et al. 1995), but in some cases one may masquerade as the other (Pennington et al. 1993). To determine whether an individual has comorbid ADHD and LD, evaluations of both are required (Fletcher et al. 1999).

The reported prevalence of the co-occurrence of ADHD and LD (see Semrud-Clikeman et al. 1992) varies widely in the literature (e.g., from 10% [Forness et al. 1992] to 90% [Silver 1981]). This wide variation is probably the result of referral patterns to practitioners with specialties that attract different types of complicated (comorbid) or uncomplicated (pure) cases. Clearly, another source of variation is the definition used for each disorder, which also produces wide variation in the estimated prevalence of separate disorders—from 1% to 20% for ADHD (see Swanson et al. 1998) and from 1% to 30% for LD (see Kavale and Forness 1996; Lerner 1993).

Some guidelines for the assessment of ADHD are provided in the practice parameters published by the American Academy of Child and Adolescent Psychiatry (AACAP) in 1991 and revised in 1997. Some guidelines for the assessment of LD are provided in the practice parameters published by the AACAP in 1998. The assessment of ADHD and LD differs in fundamental ways. The assessment battery of the Multimodal Treatment Study for ADHD (MTA Study; Hinshaw et al. 1997) provides an excellent example to highlight these differences.

The assessment of ADHD is based on psychiatric interviews and symptom rating scales. In the MTA battery, the instruments used were the Diagnostic Interview Schedule for Children (DISC-IV; Shaffer et al. 1993), which was administered to the parent, and the Swanson, Nolan, and Pelham (SNAP-IV) rating scale (Swanson 1992), which was completed by both teacher and parent. Thus, the basis for the diagnosis of ADHD is subjective assessment of behavior reported by caregivers, and no psychometric or psychological tests are generally accepted for diagnosis (Baren and Swanson 1996). In contrast, the assessment of LD does use psychometric tests of potential and achievement (American Academy of Child and Adolescent Psychiatry 1998). In the MTA battery, the assessment instruments used were the Wechsler Intelligence Scale for

Children (WISC-III; Wechsler 1991) and the Wechsler Individual Achievement Test-Screener (WIAT-S 1992). In this chapter, we describe how these specific assessment procedures for ADHD and LD were applied to evaluate the large (N = 579) MTA sample of 7- to 9-year-old children referred for ADHD. In particular, in this chapter we will illustrate one component of the assessment of LD—namely, the estimation of a discrepancy in ability and achievement. Two methods are commonly discussed and used (see Reynolds 1992): the simple difference method and the predicted achievement method. The simple difference method is based on the subtraction of achievement tests scores (e.g., reading, math reasoning, and spelling from the WIAT-S) from a measure of ability (e.g., full-scale [FS] IQ from the WISC-III). In the predicted achievement method, the IQ scores are replaced by the estimated achievement test scores predicted by the IQ scores. These predictions are based on the correlation between the ability–achievement measures and are presented in a table in the WIAT-S manual.

There are many controversies surrounding the use of discrepancy scores in the assessment of LD. First, there are questions about the validity of the discrepancy approach (see Fletcher et al. 1999; Lyon 1989; Stanovich and Segal 1994), so there is some controversy whether any discrepancy method should be used. Second, if a discrepancy approach is used, there is no consensus about which of these two methods should be adopted. The choice of one method over the other carries a bias that favors individuals with low or high IQ. Third, for both methods different statistical assumptions and formulas have been used to establish cutoffs for "significant discrepancy," and for a given statistical significance level the number of cases identified by the two methods may be very different. Therefore, we will point out at the beginning that no specific discrepancy method is endorsed here. Instead, we are providing examples of multiple methods used to characterize the baseline assessment of LD in the MTA sample, and we propose to evaluate these different approaches in the next stage of this prospective follow-up study of ADHD children.

Also, our emphasis on discrepancy methods should not be misconstrued as a primer for performing an assessment of LD or SLD. Although a discrepancy between achievement and intellectual ability may be a reasonable place to begin, a comprehensive assessment of deficits should include additional tests that measure the underlying skill deficits that cause the disorder or disability in the first place (see Lyon 1996 for a review). For example, specific tests of phonological processing can reveal skill deficits that are not revealed by common achievement tests. These skills deficits are targets for interventions in programs designed to improve reading proficiency (see Lovett et al., in press).

Current Guidelines for Educational Services

Because access to services in medicine and in education often is based on diagnosis or labeling, operational definitions have been proposed in medical manuals (e.g., DSM-IV; ICD-10 [World Health Organization 1992]) and in federal law (e.g., IDEA) and regulations (see U.S. Department of Education 1998). The histories of the definitions of ADHD and LD have been discussed in the practice parameters (American Academy of Child and Adolescent Psychiatry 1991, 1997, 1998), so only a short review is necessary here.

The current definition of ADHD in DSM-IV evolved from the definition of hyperkinetic reaction to childhood listed in DSM-II (American Psychiatric Association 1968), which was renamed attention deficit disorder (ADD) in DSM-III (American Psychiatric Association 1980) and attention-deficit hyperactivity disorder (ADHD) in DSM-III-R (American Psychiatric Association 1987). An important advance occurred in the early 1990s: after decades of differences, the specific symptoms listed in the two primary psychiatric manuals (ICD-10 and DSM-IV) converged, so now the same set of 18 are used around the world. The ADHD label was retained in DSM-IV, but some changes were made in the criteria to allow for three subtypes (inattentive, hyperactive/impulsive, and combined). In ICD-10 (World Health Organization 1992), a different label was used (hyperkinetic disorder [HKD], disturbance of activity and attention). Despite the use of the same symptoms for diagnosing ADHD and HKD, there are still differences in decision rules for making a diagnosis in the areas of subtypes and comorbid conditions, which are discouraged or not allowed by IDC-10 criteria and guidelines (see Swanson et al. 1998). The criteria in both manuals include a cutoff in terms of a "symptom count," which in DSM-IV is set at 6 (or more) of the 9 symptoms listed in either (or both) of the two domains of inattention and hyperactivity/impulsivity. However, meeting this criterion alone is not sufficient for a diagnosis. In addition, early onset (by age 7 years), impairment (in multiple settings), and long duration (chronic not episodic presence) are specified as part of the complex criteria for making a diagnosis of ADHD. Also, clinical experience and expertise is required for sophisticated evaluation of comorbid conditions and use of exclusion criteria (see Pliszka et al., in press). There are many published discussions on diagnosis of ADHD (see American Academy of Child and Adolescent Psychiatry 1998), including a detailed discussion of the diagnostic methods of the MTA study (see Hinshaw et al. 1997), so only an example (rather than another discussion) will be presented here.

The current definition of LD in DSM-IV evolved from the definitions of specific developmental disorders (DSM-III) and academic skills disorders (DSM-III-R) (see Arnold 1990). In the description of diagnostic features, the DSM-IV manual (p. 46) presents a clear position on the first controversy mentioned earlier (i.e., whether the discrepancy approach should be used or not). The manual states that learning disorders (i.e., reading disorder, mathematics disorder, and disorder of written expression) are diagnosed when achievement is ". . . substantially below that expected for age, schooling, and level of intelligence," and this produces significant interference with daily activities. The critical term "substantially below" is defined as ". . . a discrepancy of more than 2 standard deviations between achievement and IQ." Thus, the DSM-IV manual recommends the simple difference method of estimating ability–achievement discrepancy. In contrast, ICD-10 (p. 244) recommends the predicted achievement method by suggesting a comparison of actual achievement to ". . . the average expected level of achievement for any given IQ level." This is even clearer in the companion manual for diagnostic criteria for research (World Health Organization 1993, pp. 144–146), in which the guidelines specify a discrepancy cutoff ". . . that is at least 2 standard errors of prediction below the level expected on the basis of the child's chronological age and general intelligence." This DSM–ICD difference highlights the second controversy mentioned earlier in this chapter—the lack of consensus about which method should be used for estimating ability–achievement discrepancy. However, both manuals provide leeway in the application of cutoffs. DSM-IV acknowledges that a smaller discrepancy ("between 1 and 2 standard deviations") is often used when another disorder may compromise IQ and thus make it more difficult to meet the stated cutoff of 2 standard deviations. ICD-10 acknowledges that the discrepancy requirements are unlikely to be met "in routine clinical practice." So, the third controversy (i.e., the specification of cutoffs) is also reflected in clinical assessment of LD. These three controversies will be addressed in the example presented in this chapter.

As reviewed briefly in the beginning of this chapter, the IDEA uses disability categories to qualify students for services, rather than disorder categories as in DSM-IV. The disability categories that are relevant to this chapter are specific learning disability (SLD) and other health impairment (OHI). However, qualifying for the SLD or OHI disability category is not sufficient to qualify for special education services under the IDEA. Also, the severity of the disability must be evaluated to help determine whether the disability adversely affects educational performance. Carefully worded guidelines for specifying which students qualify for special education and related services are based on laws (e.g., the IDEA) and implementing regulations in the Code of Federal Regulations (CFR) (see U.S. Department of Education 1998).

The current definitions of SLD evolved from the federal definitions of handicapping conditions (National Advisory Committee on Handicapped Children 1968) that were incorporated into Public Law 91-230 (Children With Specific Learning Disabilities Act 1969). These definitions remained in the well-known Public Law 94-142 (Education for All Handicapped Children Act 1975), which was renamed the Individuals With Disabilities Education Act in 1990 and recently was reauthorized by Public Law 105-17 (IDEA Amendments 1997; Yell and Shriner 1997). The core features stated in the CFR (Title 34 §300.7(c)(10)) are essentially the same as when they were formulated in 1968: SLD is defined as "a disorder in one or more of the basic psychological processes involved in understanding or in using language, spoken or written, that may manifest itself in an imperfect ability to listen, think, speak, read, write, spell, or to do mathematical calculations, including conditions such as perceptual disabilities, brain injury, minimal brain dysfunction, dyslexia, and developmental aphasia. . . ." Two additional federal statutes cover a broader range of disabilities: the Rehabilitation Act of 1973 (section 504), a civil rights law that prohibits discrimination on the basis of disability, and the Americans With Disabilities Act of 1990 (Title II), which extends this prohibition to public entities, including school districts.

The U.S. Department of Education offers guidance about the statutes and regulations through letters and memoranda. The federal guidelines (e.g., Assistance to the States for Education of Children With Disabilities; CFR, Title 34, Part 200) specify that the assessment and review be performed by a qualified team, consisting of professionals from the school (including the teachers who know the child) as well as the parents of the child. If a disability (e.g., SLD or OHI) is verified, then this team must develop an individualized educational plan (IEP) tailored to meet the specific needs of the child. These guidelines make it clear that the label SLD refers to a complex condition that is not just one entity and that comprehensive assessment and review of each child is required to determine if a disability exists.

The interpretation of the relationship of ADHD to the disability categories in the educational statutes and regulations has been controversial. Almost a decade ago, this was clarified by a memorandum from the U.S. Department of Education (Davila et al. 1991). This memorandum was based on broad input generated by a Notice of Inquiry on ADHD (Federal Register 1990) and provided guidance on how children with ADHD could be determined eligible for services under two laws (i.e., part B of the IDEA and section 504 of the Rehabilitation Act of 1973). As specified in the 1991 memorandum, if ADHD produced "limited alertness" that seriously impaired school performance, then qualification under part B of IDEA was possible in the OHI category. In the latest statement of the regulations for IDEA (Code of Federal Regulations, March 12, 1999), "limited alertness" was defined to include a heightened alertness to environmental stimuli resulting in limited alertness to relevant stimuli in the educational setting. If the severity of impairment due to ADHD is not sufficient to qualify for SED, SLD, OHI status under educational laws, then "504" accommodations for ADHD in the regular classroom are directed by the civil rights laws.

Even though official definitions exist in psychiatric manuals for ADHD and LD, and in educational laws and regulations for OHI, SED, and SLD, the methods to identify individuals with these disorders or disabilities are controversial. Critical scientific issues have been identified in the literature. With respect to ADHD/OHI, a critical topic is the use of subjective impressions of symptoms to establish severity of disorder (National Institute of Health 1998). With respect to LD/SLD, a critical topic is the use of the ability–achievement discrepancy approach to identify these conditions and to recommend treatment (see Lyon 1989, 1996). We will address these two topics in an example based on the MTA sample of children with ADHD, and we will discuss some controversies about statistical methods that have been applied for these diagnostic purposes. SED assessment of children is not addressed here.

Methods Used in the MTA to Evaluate ADHD and LD

In the MTA, the diagnosis of ADHD was based on a broad assessment that included a structured psychiatric interview (the DISC-IV) with the child's parents. Among other criteria, the DISC-IV evaluates each of the symptoms of ADHD according to the parents' judgment about its presence or absence and provides a symptom count to determine whether DSM-IV criteria are met (i.e., the presence of at least six of the nine symptoms of inattention and at least six of the nine symptoms of hyperactivity-impulsivity). In the MTA assessment, the parent interview provided information about the child's behavior at home and at school, but the teacher was not interviewed to provide direct diagnostic information. To supplement the DISC-IV interview, the SNAP-IV was used to obtain directly from the teacher (as well as from the parent) ratings of the 18 DSM-IV symptoms of ADHD.

As shown in Table 4–1, the first 18 items on the SNAP-IV are the specific DSM-IV criteria for ADHD, and the rating categories ask for a judgment of degree of presence (not at all, just a little, pretty much, or very much). If fewer than six symptoms were endorsed on either domain on the parent DISC-IV, then a score of 2 (pretty much) or 3 (very much) on the teacher-completed SNAP-IV rating scale was taken as evidence of symptom presence for up to two additional ADHD symptoms in either domain.

Controversy exists regarding the combination of information from rating scales and structured interviews to make psychiatric diagnoses. A primary purpose of a structured interview (such as the DISC-IV) is to provide qualitative information for a categorical diagnosis (e.g., for ADHD, presence of at least six of nine symptoms of inattention and/or hyperactivity-impulsivity as stated in DSM-IV). Typically, the interview is with the parent, who conveys information about the child in the home and school setting. In contrast, a primary purpose of a rating scale is to provide quantitative information about severity of symptoms in a domain (e.g., the average rating per item on a 0–3 scale). Typically, ratings are obtained directly from two sources (parents and teachers), but there is no consensus about the rating category that denotes "presence" (see Gaub and Carlson 1997; Pelham et al. 1993; Wolraich et al. 1996) or how to combine these two sources (see Swanson et al. 1999). Despite similar content (i.e., the ADHD symptoms), the information obtained using these two methods (interviews and ratings) is not always consistent.

Even when the same method or instrument is used, information from different sources is not always consistent. This results in low parent–teacher correlation (e.g., about 0.30) of ratings of problem behaviors (see Achenbach 1987). The source differences may be partially due to situational differences in behavior rather than to deficiencies in rating scales. However, different levels of tolerance for disruptive behavior, different ulterior motives for adjusting ratings to be lower or higher, and other factors certainly contribute to low correlation of parent and teacher ratings. A brief interview with both sources about disagreements at the item level is recommended to clarify and understand the expected source differences in subjective ratings of psychopathology (see Swanson et al. 1999).

Table 4–1. Swanson, Nolan, and Pelham (SNAP-IV) rating scale

Name: _____ Gender: _____ Age: _____ Grade: _____

Ethnicity: ❑ African American ❑ Asian ❑ Caucasian ❑ Hispanic ❑ Other

For Teacher: Completed by: _____ Type of class: _____ Class size: _____

Telephone # at school: _____ Recommended times for follow-up call: _____

For Parent: Completed by: _____ # Parents living in home: _____ Family size: _____

Period of time covered by rating: ❑ Past week ❑ Past month ❑ Past year ❑ Lifetime ❑ Other

For each item, check the column that best describes this child:

	Not At All	Just A Little	Pretty Much	Very Much
1. Fails to give close attention to details or makes careless mistakes in schoolwork or tasks	___	___	___	___
2. Has difficulty sustaining attention in tasks or play activities	___	___	___	___
3. Does not seem to listen when spoken to directly	___	___	___	___
4. Does not follow through on instructions and fails to finish schoolwork, chores, or duties	___	___	___	___
5. Has difficulty organizing tasks and activities	___	___	___	___
6. Avoids, dislikes, or reluctantly engages in tasks requiring sustained mental effort	___	___	___	___
7. Loses things necessary for activities (e.g., toys, school assignments, pencils, or books)	___	___	___	___
8. Is distracted by extraneous stimuli	___	___	___	___
9. Is forgetful in daily activities	___	___	___	___

Table 4–1. Swanson, Nolan, and Pelham (SNAP-IV) rating scale *(continued)*

	Not At All	Just A Little	Pretty Much	Very Much
10. Fidgets with hands or feet or squirms in seat	—	—	—	—
11. Leaves seat in classroom or in other situations in which remaining seated is expected	—	—	—	—
12. Runs about or climbs excessively in situations in which it is inappropriate	—	—	—	—
13. Has difficulty playing or engaging in leisure activities quietly	—	—	—	—
14. Is "on the go" or often acts as if "driven by a motor"	—	—	—	—
15. Talks excessively	—	—	—	—
16. Blurts out answers before questions have been completed	—	—	—	—
17. Has difficulty awaiting turn	—	—	—	—
18. Interrupts or intrudes on others (e.g., butts into conversations/games)	—	—	—	—

For the MTA, the four-point response on the SNAP-IV was scored 0–3 (not at all = 0, just a little = 1, pretty much = 2, and very much = 3). Subscale scores were calculated by summing the scores on the items in each domain (i.e., items 1–9 for inattention and items 10–18 for hyperactivity/impulsivity) and dividing by the number of items (i.e., 9). In a local normative control group (LNCG) recruited from classmates of the MTA subjects, the 95th percentile cutoff for teacher ratings were 2.6 for inattention and 1.9 for hyperactivity/impulsivity. For parent ratings, the 95th percentile cutoffs were 1.8 for inattention and 1.3 for hyperactivity/impulsivity. In subsequent use of the SNAP-IV, the rating category "pretty much" was replaced by "quite a bit" and the word "often" was added to items to create an identical match with the DSM-IV symptom list (see Pliszka et al. 1999; Swanson et al. 1999). These changes had little impact on school-wide norms derived from teacher ratings.

For a psychiatric diagnosis of ADHD, in addition to presence, severity and impairment in at least two settings must be verified. The data from the MTA study reveal some potential problems with ratings of ADHD symptoms used for this purpose. Figures 4–1A (teacher ratings) and Figure 4–1B (parent ratings) show the distributions of ADHD symptom-severity scores in an LNCG recruited from classmates of the MTA subjects. For this control group, instead of the normal distribution (a symmetric, bell-shaped curve) the negative binomial (or "contagious poisson") distribution (a skewed, J-shaped curve) provides the best fit (see McCleary et al., unpublished observations, 2000).

As shown in Figure 4–1, almost all control children have scores less than 1.0 (i.e., ratings less than "just a little") on the SNAP-IV rating scale. This distribution of scores should be expected for any rating scale of psychopathology, in which the items are defined as problem behaviors that are not present in the vast majority of children in the general population. As a consequence, the use of usual statistics to identify the extreme upper end of the distribution (e.g., the mean ± 1.65 SD, represented by a z-score of 1.65 or the equivalent T score of 66.5) will identify more than the expected number of students with extreme scores. An evaluation of the LNCG demonstrates the impact of this in the MTA example: instead of the expected 5%, the mean ± 1.65 SD cutoff for overall severity of the 18 symptoms identified almost 10% of this sample of the 7- to 9-year-old school population in the extreme range. It is likely that the psychometric properties of any rating scale of psychopathology would have the same bias toward overidentification by statistical cutoffs. To guard against this, percentile cutoffs are recommended (see Swanson et al. 1999).

In addition to this complication about severity estimates based on norms, the use of rating scales is complicated by low correlation between parent and teacher ratings of clinical cases (see above). The differences between parents' and teachers' subjective reports of behavior contribute to a "disconnect" in the assessment of ADHD children (National Institute of Health 1998). The use of interviews to ask both sources about discrepancies has been recommended as one way to reduce this type of disconnect between home and school sources (see Swanson et al. 1999), but even then

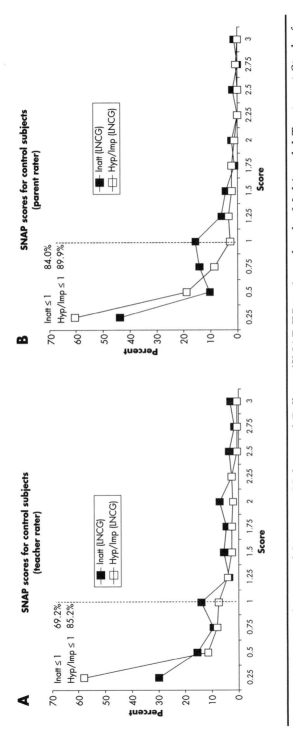

Figure 4–1. Distribution of Swanson, Nolan, and Pelham (SNAP-IV) ratings for the Multimodal Treatment Study for ADHD (MTA Study) Local Normative Control Group (LNCG). Inatt = inattention; Hyp/Imp = hyperactivity-impulsivity. These data are for 169 of the 288 LNCG subjects for whom parent and teacher ratings were available.

complete agreement is not expected due to situational differences in behavior. This is a problem because DSM-IV criteria require confirmation of symptoms in more than one setting (usually the home and school). However, no consensus exists about how to reconcile the expected differences in parent and teacher ratings. For example, use of the "and" rule (to accept as symptoms only those items with high ratings by both sources) reduces the number of cases meeting severity criteria to a very low percentage of the school-aged population (see Leung et al. 1996, 1998), whereas use of the "or" rule (to accept as symptoms all items with high ratings by either source) might increase the number of cases to an unacceptably high percentage.

In the MTA procedure, a combination of the parent interview and a partial "or" rule was used (see MTA Cooperative Group 1999a): if the DISC-IV interview identified at least 10 but fewer than 12 symptoms (because 6 are needed in each subtype: inattention or hyperactivity-impulsivity), then high teacher ratings on the SNAP-IV ("pretty much" = 2 or "very much" = 3) on up to two items not endorsed by the parents were allowed to contribute to meeting the inclusions criteria for a diagnosis of ADHD, combined type.

The use of psychometric test data to characterize the MTA sample has not been discussed in detail elsewhere, so a preview of the issues and problems is presented here. The MTA investigators decided not to engage in a formal evaluation of SLD, which is rightfully the role of a qualified team and requires the interpretation of comprehensive assessments and a review of the school history of the child. Instead, we performed one component of the assessment by applying several methods to obtain ability–achievement discrepancies that are specified in educational regulations (for SLD) and psychiatric manuals (for LD). As discussed above, a significant discrepancy alone certainly does not identify LD or SLD. For example, a clinical evaluation may override the absence of an ability–achievement discrepancy based on the impact of a comorbid condition on estimates of IQ (see DSM-IV). Also, a team evaluating a child's need for special education services may override ineligibility based on the lack of a significant discrepancy (see U.S. Department of Education 1998). In fact, this often occurs (see Gresham and Witt 1997; Mac-Millian and Speece, in press; MacMillan et al. 1996, 1998).

So, we should repeat that our example of using different ability–achievement discrepancy methods is not an endorsement of these procedures. Instead, we adopted a strategy of applying different discrepancy approaches to the MTA sample at baseline to identify subgroups that can be followed over time to evaluate the usefulness of these measures for predicting outcome or identifying moderators of treatment effects. We are aware that some critics of the discrepancy approach (e.g., see Fletcher et al. 1999) have recommended the use of low achievement alone to identifying children in need of special education services. This approach has been used alone or in combination with a discrepancy approach (see Barkley 1998; B. S. G. Molina and W. E. Pelham, unpublished observations, 2000). In follow-up investigations of the MTA sample, we will evaluate some of these alternative and/or hybrid approaches as well.

In the MTA assessment battery, we used the WISC-III to provide measures of full-scale IQ as well as subscales of verbal IQ and performance IQ. We used the WIAT-S to provide three subscales as measures of achievement (reading, math reasoning, and spelling). One reason that WISC-III and the WIAT-S were chosen for the MTA assessment battery was that their norms were collected on the same sample of cases ($n = 1,888$), which provided estimates of the correlation (r) between any two IQ and achievement measures. As discussed below, these correlations are necessary for some methods of calculating ability–achievement discrepancies.

We do realize that other achievement tests may be used more widely than the WIAT-S, as suggested by the practice parameters for learning disorders (American Academy of Child and Adolescent Psychiatry 1998). For example, the Woodcock-Johnson Psycho-Educational Battery (Woodcock and Johnson 1989) is more commonly used by schools to assess students. Also, it is perplexing that some other tests of achievement (e.g., the Wide Range Achievement Test [WRAT]) may yield substantially more cases with a significant discrepancy than the WIAT (see Bocian et al. 1999). Thus, the selection of a particular achievement test is likely to affect the magnitude of IQ–achievement discrepancies measured by the test.

After selecting the psychometric instruments, it is necessary to make another decision to select a discrepancy method. The two primary methods for calculating ability–achievement discrepancy are the simple difference method and the predicted achievement method described previously. In the WIAT-S manual, tables are provided to help the user implement either method. As amply discussed in the literature (see Reynolds 1992), the predicted achievement method and the simple difference method are based on different assumptions and expected to yield different results. In this chapter, we provide examples for both methods to show how they differ when applied to the large MTA sample.

In our example of the simple difference method, we used the standard scores for full-scale IQ and the standard scores for reading, math reasoning, and spelling from the WISC-III and WIAT-S. For both of these instruments, the scores are standardized so that the norm sample has a mean of 100 and a standard deviation of 15. According to this method, a WIAT standard score is subtracted from a WISC standard score to obtain the simple difference discrepancy. This is the method recommended in DSM-IV.

The predicted achievement method makes adjustments based on the correlation of the IQ and achievement test score, which takes into account the concept of "regression to the mean." In the WIAT-S manual, Table C.1 (p. 164) provides the predicted achievement test scores for WISC full-scale IQ values from 40 to 160. Inspection of the tabled values shows that predicted achievement is lower than IQ for above-average ability (i.e., for IQ = 115, the predicted reading achievement is 109) and higher than IQ for below-average ability (i.e., for IQ = 85, the predicted reading achievement is 91). The magnitude of the adjustment is inversely related to the correlation between IQ and the specific achievement tests, so for a given IQ smaller adjustments are made for the math reasoning subtest ($r = 0.72$) than for the reading ($r = 0.60$) or spelling ($r = 0.52$) subtests of the WIAT-S.

After an ability–achievement discrepancy is calculated, either by the simple difference method (IQ minus actual achievement) or by the predicted achievement method (predicted achievement minus actual achievement), it is compared with a cutoff value. In the WIAT-S manual, cutoff values are provided in Table C.4 (for the predicted achievement method) and Table C.6 (for the simple difference method). The statistical assumptions and formulas used to establish the cutoffs in Tables C.4 and C.6 are different for the two methods (see pp. 80–81 of the WIAT-S manual). Because these procedures are complex and have been discussed elsewhere (Reynolds 1992) and in the WIAT manual, only the results (in terms of relative magnitude of the cutoffs for the two methods) are discussed here.

The entries in Tables C.4 and C.6 provide the magnitude of discrepancies that are required for statistical significance for P values of 0.05 and 0.01. The cutoffs vary somewhat across age (due to slightly different correlations in the norm sample), but each table provides an average cutoff summarizing the effects across age. The two methods have very different cutoffs for the reading and spelling subtests, but not for the math reasoning subtest. For example, the $P = 0.01$ cutoffs for the predicted achievement method (see WIAT-S, Table C.4) are 20.60 for reading, 20.74 for spelling, and only 13.59 for math reasoning. In contrast, for the simple difference method (see WIAT-S, Table C.6) the cutoffs for significant discrepancies are lower for reading (13.78) and spelling (15.09) but higher for math reasoning (15.56).

In our example, we noticed several peculiarities in the WIAT-S manual and procedures that deserve mention but not detailed discussion in this chapter. First, we noticed that the headings of the two crucial tables (C.4 and C.6) mistakenly included a reference to a "composite score." This apparently was a mistake made when the heading from the complete WIAT manual was duplicated in the WIAT-S manual, but the naïve user should be warned to avoid confusion. Second, we noticed that the relationship among the WIAT subtests was different for the two methods, primarily due to the math reasoning subtest (which for the predicted achievement method had lower cutoff values than reading or spelling but for the simple difference method had higher values). We investigated this and decided it was due to the combination of two psychometric properties of the WIAT, both of which are incorporated into the formula for calculating a cutoff for the predicted achievement method: the correlation with IQ (which for math reasoning was the highest correlation of the three WIAT subtests) and the test–retest reliability (which for math reasoning was the lowest). Both of these relationships operated to reduce the relative size of the math reasoning cutoff when applying the formula for the predicted achievement method but not for the simple difference method. This is an interesting statistical-methodological point about the predicted achievement method, which we plan to discuss in more detail elsewhere.

An Example From the MTA Study

The assessment of the MTA sample provided IQ and achievement scores for more than 500 children with ADHD, combined type. We use this sample to provide examples of the simple difference and the predicted achievement methods for estimating ability–achievement discrepancies. In Figure 4–2, we present the distributions of scores from the WISC IQ tests (on the left) and the WIAT-S achievement tests scores (on the right) for the MTA sample. These data are for 7- to 9-year-old children with ADHD, combined type, and scores were available on 525 of the 579 individuals in the sample.

The three graphs on the left show that the distributions of IQ scores for the MTA sample are approximately normal. The slight rightward skewness was most likely due to an exclusion criterion that set the lower bound of 80 on at least one of the IQ measures, unless overridden by a higher score on the Scales of Independent Behavior (SIB) (Bruininks et al. 1985). Full-scale, verbal, and performance IQ all were slightly (but not significantly) above the expected mean (about 100) with the expected SD (about 15). Thus, the MTA sample provides a large group of children with normal ability for this example on discrepancy analysis.

The three graphs on the right show the distributions for the three WIAT subtests. In the MTA sample, these distributions had slightly lower means than the IQ distributions and slightly greater rightward skewness. In the graphs, the cases identified by low achievement (85 or less) are shaded: about 20% ($n = 104$) had low reading scores, about 17% ($n = 88$) had low math scores, and about 23% ($n = 124$) had low spelling scores. When all three tests were considered, 32.8% of the sample had a low achievement test score on at least one subtest of the WIAT. These are the cases that would be identified for special services by the "low achievement" criteria that have been recommended for use instead of the discrepancy approach (see Fletcher et al. 1999).

In Figure 4–3, we present the distributions of the discrepancies for the predicted achievement method (on the left) and the simple difference method (on the right). These distributions are quite similar for the two methods, which is expected. For both methods the mean discrepancy is positive (from 2.74 to 9.92 points), indicating slight underachievement for the overall group.

For both methods, the $P = 0.05$ and $P = 0.01$ cutoff values (taken from Tables C.4 and C.6) are shown in the graphs for reading, math reasoning, and spelling. Despite the similarity of the distributions of discrepancies for the two methods, the percentages of the MTA sample with "significant discrepancies" are very different for the reading and spelling subtests of the WIAT-S. For these two achievement tests, the simple difference method identifies about twice as many children with significant discrepancies as the predicted achievement method. The relative difference is larger for the strict ($P = 0.01$) cutoffs (close to 28% vs. 11% for both reading and spelling) than for the $P = 0.05$ cutoffs (close to 36% vs. 19%). These large differences are due to different magnitudes of the cutoffs, not to differences in the distributions of discrepancies. On the math reasoning test, the percentages of the MTA sample exceeding the cutoffs are about the same for the two methods (22% vs. 18% for the $P = 0.05$ cutoffs and 14% vs. 13% for the $P = 0.01$ cutoffs).

To relate these groups of ADHD cases with "significant discrepancies" to the group with low achievement, we calculated the number of cases with low achievement (using 85 as the cutoff) that also had significant discrepancies with low or high achievement. Surprisingly, more low-achievement cases were identified by the simple difference method than the predicted achievement method for the reading and spelling subtests. For the $P = 0.05$ cutoffs, out of the 104 cases with low reading achievement, the simple difference method identified 58 and the predicted achievement method identified 45; for the 124 cases with low spelling achievement, the simple difference method identified 65 and the predicted achievement method identified 60. In contrast, for the 88 cases with low math reasoning achievement, the simple difference method identified only 27, whereas the predicted achievement

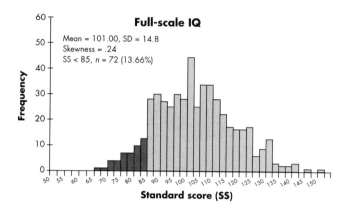

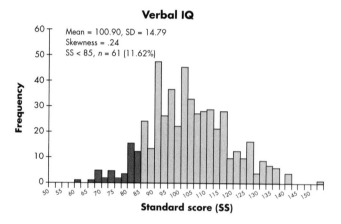

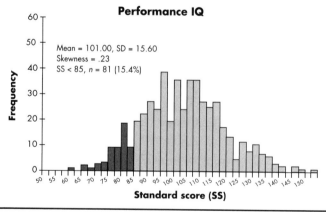

Figure 4–2. Distributions of WISC-III IQ scores (left) and WIAT-S

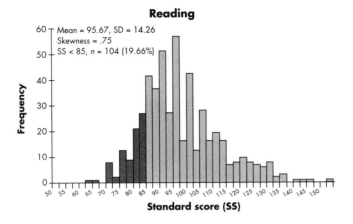

Reading

Mean = 95.67, SD = 14.26
Skewness = .75
SS < 85, n = 104 (19.66%)

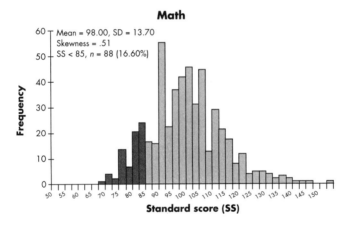

Math

Mean = 98.00, SD = 13.70
Skewness = .51
SS < 85, n = 88 (16.60%)

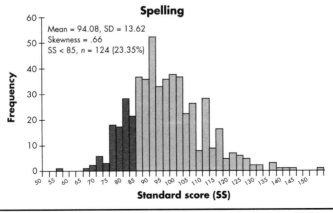

Spelling

Mean = 94.08, SD = 13.62
Skewness = .66
SS < 85, n = 124 (23.35%)

achievement test scores (right) for the MTA sample.

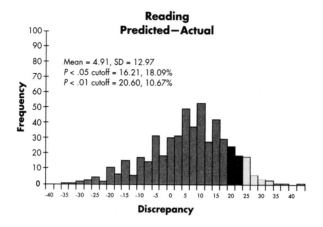

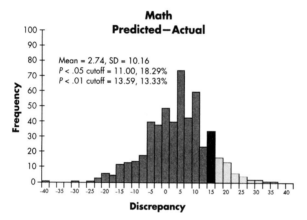

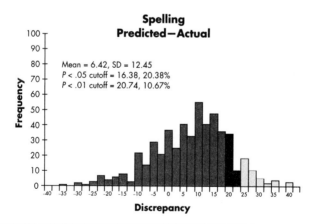

Figure 4–3. Distributions of the predicted achievement discrepancies and

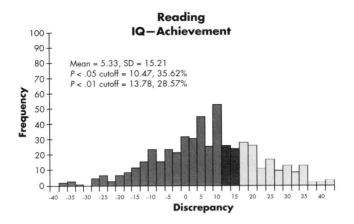

Reading
IQ—Achievement

Mean = 5.33, SD = 15.21
$P < .05$ cutoff = 10.47, 35.62%
$P < .01$ cutoff = 13.78, 28.57%

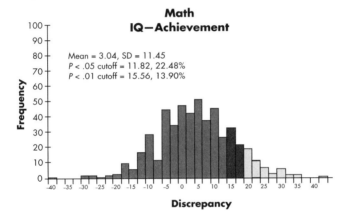

Math
IQ—Achievement

Mean = 3.04, SD = 11.45
$P < .05$ cutoff = 11.82, 22.48%
$P < .01$ cutoff = 15.56, 13.90%

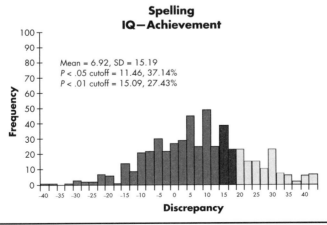

Spelling
IQ—Achievement

Mean = 6.92, SD = 15.19
$P < .05$ cutoff = 11.46, 37.14%
$P < .01$ cutoff = 15.09, 27.43%

simple difference discrepancies in the MTA sample.

method identified 41. The number of low achievement cases identified by these cutoffs depended on the placement of the cutoffs by the assumptions and formula by the two methods (as discussed above) as well as by the adjustments based on predicted achievement (which depended on the correlation of IQ with the different subtests).

The use of the WIAT spelling subtest is problematic (Kavale and Forness 1996), because a discrepancy in spelling alone does not meet the IDEA eligibility criteria for SLD. Often, just the reading and math reasoning are considered to see how many children in a sample would have a significant discrepancy in either of these two tests. We calculated the percentage of cases exceeding the cutoff on either the reading or math reasoning discrepancy for both ability–achievement discrepancy methods. The percentages were higher for the simple difference method than for predicted achievement method for the $P = 0.05$ cutoffs (28.8% vs. 41.1%) and the $P = 0.01$ cutoffs (32.6% vs. 18.5%).

The cutoffs for the predicted achievement method and the simple difference method are based on very different assumptions, and this makes it difficult to compare the overall number or percentage of cases identified by these methods. To put these methods on an equal footing, the percentile cutoffs shown in Tables C.5 and C.7 in the WIAT-S manual can be used. The magnitude of the cutoff values provided for these two tables is similar (for 1% of the population, standard score differences of 23, 21, and 25 for the predicted achievement method and 29, 24, and 31 for the simple difference method; for 5% of the population, 16, 15, and 17 for the predicted achievement method and 18, 17, and 21 for the simple difference method). A comparison of Tables C.5 and C.7 indicates that the percentile cutoffs for the simple difference method are larger than for the predicted achievement method—the opposite of the comparison of the two methods based on the statistical cutoff values given in Tables C.4 and C.6.

Discussion

This example from the MTA study provides some information that might be relevant for the psychiatrist performing an assessment of ADHD and LD according to the criteria in DSM-IV. The results have implications for the use of both rating scales and psychometric tests in the assessment of children with ADHD and LD.

First, the assessment of the MTA control group (the LNCG) provided norms for assessing the severity of ADHD symptoms. In the MTA example, we demonstrated that the ratings of symptom severity (by parents and teachers) in the LNCG were not normally distributed. If statistical applications assuming a normal distribution were used with these norms, the severity of ADHD relative to the control population would be overestimated. Thus, this example from the MTA demonstrates how the use of rating scales alone could result in overidentification of extreme cases, and we recommended the use of percentile cutoffs to avoid this statistical artifact. Of course, the MTA assessment procedure did not rely on ratings of symptoms alone. We used other methods in addition to a symptom rating scale (e.g., telephone screening, the DISC-IV interview, a clinical review) to assess symptoms of ADHD. The broad and rigorous assessment clearly prevented overidentification in this sample: in the assessment of the MTA cases at baseline on the SNAP-IV, the average severity was well beyond the 95th percentiles established for the LNCG. However, our example stands as a warning against the use of a rapid, limited assessment based on rating scales alone, which may seem attractive in the climate of managed care that drives the search for efficiency. Such a limited assessment could produce false efficiency due to overidentification.

Second, the MTA example presented here provides some needed information about the percentage of ADHD children with significant ability–achievement discrepancies. The sparseness of data on this topic is shown in the WIAT-S manual, which presents information on an extremely small and not-well-documented sample of 22 children with ADHD who were evaluated with the WISC-III and WIAT-S. Based on the use of the predicted achievement method and the $P = 0.05$ cutoffs, half of this sample ($11/22 = 50\%$) had at least one significant discrepancy on the WIAT-S subtests. When the same procedures were used with the MTA sample, only a third of this larger and well-characterized sample ($178/529 = 33.9\%$) had at least one significant discrepancy. This lower percentage is consistent with a recent report by Molina and Pelham (B. S. G. Molina and W. E. Pelham, unpublished observations, 2000) of assessment of LD in a clinical sample of 109 ADHD children being followed to track substance abuse. Of course, multiple factors could account for differences across these ADHD samples, including the subtypes of ADHD in the sample, the referral sources that contributed cases to the sample, and other factors (see Semrud-Clikeman et al. 1992). However, the characteristics of the MTA sample (e.g., operational definitions of ADHD and LD, a broad recruitment strategy, large size) provide an improved estimate of comorbidity of these two conditions. This may have some practical significance for predicting the percentage of follow-up assessments of LD that may be required in a clinical sample of ADHD children.

Third, the application of different ability–achievement discrepancy methods in the large MTA sample provides an empirical basis for demonstrating differences between the methods. The simple difference method (which is recommended in DSM-IV) yielded a higher percentage of cases with significant discrepancies than the predicted achievement method (which is recommended in ICD-10). The difference was large: when all three subtests of the WIAT-S were considered using the $P = 0.05$ cutoffs (as in the example above), 46.5% of the MTA sample had at least one significant discrepancy by the simple difference method compared with 33.9% for the predicted achievement method. Thus, a psychiatrist should be aware that the diagnosis of comorbid LD might be increased by over 30% if the simple difference method is used instead of the predicted achievement method. This difference may contribute to the lower rates of comorbidity of disorders expected from ICD-10 criteria than from DSM-IV criteria (see Swanson et al. 1998). In addition, the choice of method sets a policy that affects which ADHD cases may receive a comorbid diagnosis of LD: the predicted achievement method carries a bias in favor of the low IQ cases and the simple difference method carries a bias in favor of the high IQ cases. When used in the assessment of SLD for access to special education services, both of these "method biases" should be recognized by a sophisticated child assessment team, so recommendations to the schools based on a clinical assessment of psychiatric disorders should take these factors into account.

Fourth, as discussed in the literature (Fletcher et al. 1999; Lyon 1989; Stanovich and Segal 1994), the validity of discrepancy analysis to identify LD/SLD has not been established, despite its prominent place in psychiatric manuals for evaluation of LD and educational regulations for identification of SLD. In the MTA example, about 33% of the sample had at least one low-achievement test score (defined by a cutoff of 85)—about the same percentage of the MTA sample with at least one significant discrepancy using the predicted achievement method with a $P = 0.05$ cutoff. However, the children identified by these two approaches were not the same. The prospective nature of the MTA study will provide a way to perform a rigorous test of usefulness of the low achievement method, as well as different ability–achievement discrepancy methods when applied to assess ADHD and LD in a large sample of children with ADHD. The evaluation of the MTA sample over time may prove to be a rich source of information about the school-based identification of disabilities in children with ADHD. We plan to collect information on eligibility classifications (SLD, OHI, or other categories) determined by the schools, the nature of special education services received, and the successes and difficulties in academic and social domains and to use this information to evaluate the different methods for defining comorbid ADHD and LD.

Fifth, the MTA example can provide some information on treatment effects on academic achievement as well as LD status. For example, the primary analyses (MTA Cooperative Group 1999a) revealed that on measures of WIAT-S reading, combined treatment was significantly better than either unimodal treatment over the 14-month phase of intensive intervention. However, in the companion moderator analyses (MTA Cooperative Group 1999b), there was no evidence that this treatment response was different for subgroups defined by LD status at baseline. Because the full MTA assessment battery was repeated at the end of treatment, the impact of interventions on LD status could be evaluated. L. Hechtman and colleagues (unpublished observations, 2000) reported that the systematic MTA treatments reduced ability–achievement discrepancies more than the varied and unsupervised interventions provided in the community. Further follow-up is planned, which could provide some crucial information about the long-term impact of comorbid LD on pharmacological, psychosocial, or combined treatment of children with ADHD.

Acknowledgments

The MTA Study (Multimodal Treatment Study for ADHD) is a cooperative treatment study performed by six independent research teams in collaboration with the staff of the Division of Clinical and Treatment Research of the National Institute of Mental Health (NIMH), Rockville, MD, and the Office of Special Education Programs (OSEP) of the U.S. Department of Education (DOE). The NIMH principal collaborators are Peter S. Jensen, M.D.; L. Eugene Arnold, M.D., M.Ed.; John E. Richters, Ph.D.; Joanne B. Severe, M.S.; Donald Vereen, M.D.; and Benedetto Vitiello, M.D. Principal investigators and coinvestigators from the six sites are as follows: University of California at Berkeley/San Francisco (UO1 MH50461): Stephen P. Hinshaw, Ph.D.; Glen R. Elliott, M.D., Ph.D.; Duke University (UO1 MH50447): C. Keith Conners, Ph.D.; Karen C. Wells, Ph.D.; John S. March, M.D., M.P.H.; University of California at Irvine/Los Angeles (UO1 MH50440): James M. Swanson, Ph.D.; Dennis P. Cantwell, M.D.; Timothy Wigal, Ph.D.; Long Island Jewish Medical Center/Montreal Children's Hospital (UO1 MH50453): Howard B. Abikoff, Ph.D.; Lily Hechtman, M.D.; New York State Psychiatric Institute/Columbia University/Mount Sinai Medical Center (UO1 MH50454): Laurence L. Greenhill, M.D.; Jeffrey H. Newcorn, M.D.; University of Pittsburgh (UO1 MH50467): William E. Pelham, Ph.D.; Betsy Hoza, Ph.D. Helena C. Kraemer, Ph.D. (Stanford University), was the statistical and design consultant. The OSEP/DOE principal collaborators are Lou Danielson, Ph.D., and Tom V. Hanley, Ed.D. In the previously published methodology papers for the MTA, the treatment assignments were called medication (Med), psychosocial treatment (PS), combined treatment (CT), and community-treatment assessment and referral (A&R). To more accurately reflect the actual treatments, the labels will be changed for all outcome papers to medication management (MedMgt), behavioral treatment (Beh), combined treatment (Comb), and community comparison (CC).

References

Achenbach TM, Verhulst FC, Baron GD, et al: Epidemiological comparisons of American and Dutch children, I: behavioral/emotional problems and competencies reported by parents for ages 4 to 16. J Am Acad Child Adolesc Psychiatry 26:317–325, 1987

American Academy of Child and Adolescent Psychiatry: Practice parameters for the assessment and treatment of attention-deficit hyperactivity disorder. J Am Acad Child Adolesc Psychiatry 30:I–III, 1991a

American Academy of Child and Adolescent Psychiatry: Practice parameters for the assessment and treatment of children, adolescents, and adults with attention-deficit/hyperactivity disorder. J Am Acad Child Adolesc Psychiatry 36 (suppl):85S–121S, 1997

American Academy of Child and Adolescent Psychiatry: Practice parameters for the assessment and treatment of children and adolescents with language and learning disorders. J Am Acad Child Adolesc Psychiatry 37 (suppl):46S–62S, 1998

American Psychiatric Association: Diagnostic and Statistical Manual of Mental Disorders, 2nd Edition. Washington, DC, American Psychiatric Association, 1968

American Psychiatric Association: Diagnostic and Statistical Manual of Mental Disorders, 3rd Edition. Washington, DC, American Psychiatric Association, 1980

American Psychiatric Association: Diagnostic and Statistical Manual of Mental Disorder, 3rd Edition, Revised. Washington, DC, American Psychiatric Association, 1987

American Psychiatric Association: Diagnostic and Statistical Manual of Mental Disorders, 4th Edition. Washington, DC, American Psychiatric Association, 1994

Arnold E: Learning disorders, in Psychiatric Disorders in Children and Adolescents. Edited by Garfinkel BD, Carlson GA, Weller EB. Philadelphia, PA, WB Saunders, 1990

Baren M, Swanson JM: How not to diagnose ADHD. Contemporary Pediatrics 13:53–64, 1996

Bocian K, Beebe-Frankenberger M, MacMillan DL, et al: Competing paradigms in learning disabilities classification by schools and the variations in the meaning of discrepant achievement. Learning Disabilities Research and Practice 14:1–14, 1999

Bruininks RH, Woodcock RW, Weatherman RF, et al: Scales of Independent Behavior, Examiner's Manual. Chicago, IL, Riverside, 1985

Cantwell DP, Baker L: Attention deficit disorder with and without hyperactivity: a review and comparison of matched groups. J Am Acad Child Adolesc Psychiatry 31:432–438, 1992

Davila RR, Williams ML, MacDonald JT: Clarification of Policy to Address the Needs of Children With Attention Deficit Hyperactivity Disorders Within General and/or Special Education. Memorandum from the U.S. Department of Education, Office of Special Education and Rehabilitative Services, Washington, DC, 1991

Faraone SV, Biederman J, Lehman BK, et al: Evidence for the independent familial transmission of attention deficit hyperactivity disorder and learning disabilities: results from a family genetic study. Am J Psychiatry 150:891–895, 1993

Felton RH, Wood FB: Cognitive deficits in reading disability and attention deficit disorder. J Learn Disabil 22:3–13, 1989

Fletcher JM, Shaywitz SE, Shaywitz BA: Comorbidity of learning and attention disorders: separate but equal, in Pediatric Clinics of North America, Vol 46. Edited by Morgan AM. Philadelphia, PA, WB Saunders, 1999, pp 885–897

Forness SR, Swanson JM, Cantwell DP, et al: Response to stimulant medication across six measures of school-related performance in children with ADHD and disruptive behavior. Behavioral Disorders 18:42–53, 1992

Gaub M, Carlson CL: Behavioral characteristics of DSM-IV ADHD subtypes in a school-based population. J Abnorm Child Psychol 25:103-111, 1997

Gresham FM, Witt JC: Utility of intelligence tests for treatment learning, classification, and placement decisions: recent empirical findings and future directions. School Psychology Quarterly 12:249-226, 1997

Hinshaw SP, March JS, Abikoff H, et al: Comprehensive assessment of childhood attention-deficit hyperactivity disorder in the context of a multisite, multimodal clinical trial. Journal of Attention Disorders 1:217–234, 1997

Kavale KA, Forness SR: Social skill deficits and learning disabilities: a meta-analysis. J Learn Disabil 29:226-237, 1996

Lerner JW: Learning Disabilities: Theories, Diagnosis, and Teaching Strategies, 6th Edition. Boston, MA, Houghton Mifflin, 1993

Leung PWL, Luk SL, Ho TP, et al: The diagnosis and prevalence of hyperactivity in Chinese schoolboys. Br J Psychiatry 168:486-496, 1996

Leung PWL, Connolly KJ: Attentional difficulties in hyperactive and conduct-disordered children: a processing deficit. J Child Psychol Psychiatry 35:1229-1245, 1998

Lovett MW, Steinbach KA, Frijters JC: Remediating the core deficits of developmental reading disability: a double deficit perspective. J Learn Disabil (in press)

Lyon GR: IQ is irrelevant to the definition of learning disabilities: a position in search of logic and data. J Learn Disabil 22:504–506, 512, 1989

Lyon GR: Learning disabilities, in Child Psychopathology. Edited by Mash EJ, Barkley RA. New York, Guilford, 1996, pp 390–435

MacMillan DL, Gresham FM, Siperstein GN, et al: The labyrinth of IDEA: school decisions on referred students with subaverage general intelligence. Am J Ment Retard 101:161–174, 1996

MacMillan DL, Gresham FM, Bocian KM: Discrepancy between definitions of learning disabilities and school practices: an empirical investigation. J Learn Disabil 31:314–326, 1998

MacMillan DL, Speece D: Utility of current diagnostic categories for research and practice, in Developmental Perspectives on Children With High Incidence Disabilities. Edited by Gallimore R, Bernheimer L, MacMillan D, et al. Mahwah, NJ, Lawrence Erlbaum (in press)

MTA Cooperative Group: A 14-month randomized clinical trial of treatment strategies for attention deficit hyperactivity disorder. Arch Gen Psychiatry 56:1073–1108, 1999a

MTA Cooperative Group: Moderators and mediators of treatment response for children with attention-deficit/hyperactivity disorder. Arch Gen Psychiatry 56:1088–1109, 1999b

National Advisory Committee on Handicapped Children: Special Education for Handicapped Children, First Annual Report. Washington, DC, U.S. Department of Health, Education, and Welfare, 1968

National Institutes of Health: Consensus Development Conference on Diagnosis and Treatment of Attention Deficit Hyperactivity Disorder (ADHD). Bethesda, MD, National Institutes of Health, 1998

Pennington BF, Groisser D, Welsh MC: Contrasting cognitive deficits in attention deficit hyperactivity disorder versus reading disability. Dev Psychol 29:511–523, 1993

Pliszka SR, Greenhill LL, Crimson ML, et al: The Texas Childhood Medication Algorithm Project: report of the Texas Consensus Conference Panel on Medication Treatment of Childhood Attention Deficit Hyperactivity Disorder. J Am Acad Child Adolesc Psychiatry (in press)

Reynolds CR: Two key concepts in the diagnosis of learning disabilities and the habilitation of learning. Learning Disability Quarterly 15:2–12, 1992

Semrud-Clikeman M, Biederman J, Sprich-Buckminster S, et al: Comorbidity between ADDH and learning disability: a review and report in a clinically referred sample. J Am Acad Child Adolesc Psychiatry 31:439–448, 1992

Shaffer D, Fisher P, Dulcan MK, et al: The NIMH Diagnostic Interview Schedule for Child Version 2.3 (DISC-2.3): description, acceptability, prevalence rates, and performance in the Meca Study. J Am Acad Child Adolesc Psychiatry 35:865–877, 1993

Shaywitz BA, Fletcher JM, Shaywitz SE: Defining and classifying learning disabilities and attention-deficit/hyperactivity disorder. J Child Neurol 10 (suppl 1):S50–S57, 1995

Silver LB: The relationship between learning disabilities, hyperactivity, distractibility, and behavioral problems: a clinical analysis. J Am Acad Child Psychiatry 20:385–397, 1981

Stanovich KE, Siegel LS: Phenotypic performance profiles of children with reading disabilities: a regression-based test of the phonological-core variable difference model. J Educ Psychol 86:24-25, 1994

Swanson J: School-Based Assessments and Interventions for ADD Students. Irvine, CA, KC Publishing, 1992

Swanson JM, Sergeant JA, Taylor E, et al: Attention-deficit hyperactivity disorder and hyperkinetic disorder. Lancet 351:429–433, 1998

Swanson JM, Lerner M, March J, et al: Assessment and intervention for ADHD in the schools: lessons from the MTA Study, in Pediatric Clinics of North America, Vol 46. Edited by Morgan AM. Philadelphia, PA, WB Saunders, 1999, pp 993–1009

U.S. Department of Education: Twentieth Annual Report to Congress on the Implementation of the Individuals With Disabilities Education Act. Washington, DC, Office of Special Education Program, 1998

Wechsler D: Wechsler Intelligence Scale for Children (WISC-III). San Antonio, TX, Psychological Corporation, 1991

Wechsler D: WIAT Manual: Wechsler Individual Achievement Test. San Antonio, TX, Psychological Corporation, 1992

Woodcock RW, Johnson MB: The Woodcock-Johnson Psycho-Educational Battery, Revised. Allen, TX, DLM Teaching Resources, 1989

World Health Organization: The ICD-10 Classification of Mental and Behavioral Disorders: Clinical Descriptions and Diagnostic Guidelines. Geneva, Switzerland, World Health Organization, 1992

World Health Organization: International Classification of Mental and Behavioral Disorders: Diagnostic Criteria for Research, 10th Revision. Geneva, Switzerland, World Health Organization, 1993

Yell ML, Shriner JG: The IDEA amendments of 1997: implications for special and general education teachers, administration, and teacher trainers. Focus Exceptional Child 30:1–20, 1997

Chapter 5

Language, Reading, and Motor Control Problems in ADHD

A Potential Behavioral Phenotype

Rosemary Tannock, Ph.D.

Attention-deficit/hyperactivity disorder (ADHD) frequently is associated with problems in various neurodevelopmental domains, such as speech, language, motor skills, and academic functioning (e.g., reading, spelling, arithmetic) in addition to the core behavioral symptoms of inattention and/or hyperactivity-impulsivity (Cantwell and Baker 1991; Denckla et al. 1985; Hinshaw 1992; Landgren et al. 1996; Piek et al. 1999; Tannock and Brown, in press; Tannock and Schachar 1996). These problems may be sufficiently severe and impairing to meet the diagnostic criteria for one or more of the following disorders differentiated by DSM-IV (American Psychiatric Association 1994) or the equivalent category in ICD-10 (World Health Organization 1992): communication disorders, learning disorders, or motor skills disorder. How are we to account for the complex interrelationships among all of these domains of difficulty, which are conceptualized currently as distinct disorders with implied differences in etiology and treatment requirements?

Historically, these various developmental problems, including attention and behavior problems, were grouped under the um-

This work was supported in part by a Medical Research Council of Canada Scientist Salary Award and project grants from the Medical Research Council of Canada (MT 13366) and National Institutes of Health (HD31714).

brella term *minimal brain dysfunction* (MBD) (Clements 1966). Because of the lack of empirical evidence of central nervous system (CNS) dysfunction, the concept of MBD fell into disrepute, and the various domains of dysfunction were identified and given separate diagnostic definitions (reviewed by Kalverboer 1993; Rispens and Yperen 1997; Schachar 1986). Four major areas of dysfunction previously subsumed under the term MBD have been investigated: 1) disruptive behavior problems, such as ADHD, oppositional defiant disorder (ODD), and conduct disorder; 2) communication problems, such as receptive and/or expressive language disorder; 3) learning problems, including dyslexia (reading disorder), dyscalculia (mathematics disorder), and disorder of written expression; and 4) motor control problems, such as developmental coordination disorder.

Several critical findings have emerged from empirical investigation of the four separate areas. First, epidemiological and clinical studies indicate that each of these clinical entities is prevalent and causes marked impairment (e.g., Bird et al. 1988; C. Gillberg et al. 1982; Landgren et al. 1996; Lewis et al. 1994; S. E. Shaywitz et al. 1990; Szatmari et al. 1989). Second, each of the clinical conditions shows marked heterogeneity, with marked overlap of problems both within and across each of these domains. For example, children with ADHD frequently have comorbid ODD or conduct disorder; reading disorder frequently co-occurs with mathematics disorder and disorder of written expression; ADHD frequently co-occurs with learning disorders and communication disorders; and developmental coordination disorder is often associated with specific language-learning disorders, attention and behavior problems, and visuoperceptual problems (e.g., Cantwell and Baker 1991; Denckla et al. 1985; Fletcher-Flinn et al. 1997; Kadesjo and Gillberg 1998, 1999; Ludlow et al. 1983; Wolff et al. 1995, 1996). Third, each domain of dysfunction has been found to persist into adolescence and adulthood (albeit with age-related changes in its manifestation) and to continue to show marked co-occurrence with the other domains (e.g., Bruck 1992; Caspi et al. 1996; Hellgren et al. 1994; Losse et al. 1991; Wagner et al. 1994; Weiss and Hechtman 1993). Finally, each domain of dysfunction exhibits overlapping patterns of familiality (e.g., Landgren et al.

1998; Wolff et al. 1995, 1996) with at least preliminary evidence of heritability and an association with genetic factors (e.g., Bishop et al. 1995; Cardon et al. 1994; Cook et al. 1995; Grigorenko et al. 1997; LaHoste et al. 1996; Smith et al. 1994; Swanson et al. 1998; Wolff and Melngailis 1994).

In this chapter, I focus on the complex interrelationships among ADHD, communication disorders, reading disorder, and developmental coordination disorder. I also address the considerable overlap between ADHD and the combination of deficits in attention, motor control, and perception (termed *DAMP*) that is recognized in Nordic countries. A comprehensive review of each of these domains and their overlap with ADHD is beyond the scope of this chapter; readers are referred to existing reviews (e.g., Bishop 1992; Cantwell and Baker 1991; Rasmussen and Gillberg 1999; Tannock and Schachar 1996). Rather, following a comment on several critical characteristics of ADHD and possible explanations for the observed co-occurrence of ADHD and these developmental problems, I summarize the extent and nature of the overlap of language, reading, and motor control impairments in ADHD. Next, the effect of stimulants on these associated problems is reviewed. Finally, in this chapter, I consider whether cerebellar dysfunction could be a possible explanation for the overlap of inattention/hyperactivity, speech/language problems, reading difficulties, and motor control problems and whether this constellation of problems reflects a behavioral phenotype.

Reflection on Two Critical Characteristics of ADHD: Variability and Comorbidity

The defining behavioral characteristics of inattention and hyperactivity-impulsivity in ADHD have been well documented (e.g., American Psychiatric Association 1994; World Health Organization 1992). By contrast, the most salient characteristic of *variability* or rapid fluctuation of these behavioral symptoms over time and across situations has received scant attention. For example, the most hyperactive child can be transformed suddenly into a lethargic, silent, hypoactive youngster when confronted with tasks requiring sustained concentration and effort, but he or she then races noisily out of the room when given permission to go to the washroom or watch television. Ironically, the critical thresholds for determining symptom presence and severity have been criticized because they are expressed by imprecise terms such as *often, frequently,* or *pretty much,* without further specification. Yet these terms capture precisely the essence of ADHD—variability in symptom expression.

In addition to the behavior problems, a wide range of neuropsychological deficits have been documented in ADHD, particularly in higher-order executive functions associated with control of motor responses (planning, inhibition) and working memory (e.g., Oosterlaan et al. 1998; Pennington and Ozonoff 1996; see also Purvis and Tannock 2000). Impairments are evident on tasks that require seemingly very different types of processing: those that require fast and accurate processing of information (e.g., Continuous Performance Test, stop-signal paradigm) and those that require slow and careful processing (e.g., paired associative learning tasks). Moreover, the terms *impairment* and *deficit* typically refer to inefficient performance, not to an incapacity. Inefficient performance, as reflected by *slow, highly variable,* and *inaccurate response latencies,* is one of the most robust findings in cognitive studies of ADHD across different tasks, laboratories, and cultures (Tannock, in press [NIH Consensus]). This cognitive profile is inconsistent with the common clinical assumption that ADHD is associated with a fast, careless, and impulsive style of responding.

A comment on the prevalence of comorbidity in ADHD also is warranted. The phenomenon of comorbidity raises concerns about possible weaknesses in the current nosological systems (Caron and Rutter 1991; Nottelman and Jensen 1995). Several competing hypotheses have been proposed as general explanations for comorbidity between disorders (e.g., Caron and Rutter 1991; Rutter 1994) and also as specific explanations for mechanisms linking language or reading disorder and behavior disorders (e.g., Prizant et al. 1990; Rutter and Lord 1987; Stevenson 1996). Various approaches can be used to test these competing hypotheses for comorbidity and determine whether some "comorbid patterns" in fact reflect a new diagnostic entity, heretofore unrecognized (for further discussion of this issue, see Jensen et al. 1997; Caron and Rutter 1991).

High rates of comorbidity with both internalizing and externalizing disorders are observed in community-derived and population-based samples of individuals with ADHD, as well as in clinical samples (reviewed by Biederman et al. 1991; Jensen et al. 1997). Based on a systematic review of the literature and application of specified validational criteria, Jensen and colleagues (1997) concluded that two new subclassifications of ADHD were warranted: ADHD, aggressive type, and ADHD, anxious type. In contrast, this approach could not be applied to the comorbidity between ADHD and language-learning disorders because of a lack of data (Biederman et al. 1991; Jensen et al. 1997). Moreover, although the "validation approach" may work well for evaluation of comorbid patterns with two disorders (e.g., ADHD and conduct disorder, ADHD and anxiety), its application to complex comorbid patterns (e.g., inattention/hyperactivity, language impairment, reading disorder, motor control problems) presents a challenge.

As a first step toward addressing this complex comorbidity between ADHD, language impairment, reading disorder, and developmental coordination disorder, in the following section, I review the prevalence and nature of the overlap between and among these various clinical conditions and their response to stimulant treatment.

Language Impairments Associated With ADHD

Communication disorder (also known as speech/language impairments) is an umbrella term that refers to a failure of normal speech and/or language development that cannot be explained in terms of mental or physical handicap, hearing loss, emotional disorder, or environmental deprivation (Bishop 1992). Several epidemiological and clinical studies of children with psychiatric disorders and children with language impairments have suggested an association between ADHD and language impairments (Beitchman et al. 1986; Cantwell and Baker 1987, 1991; Gualtieri et al. 1983). Results from these studies not only indicate a high degree of overlap between psychiatric disorders and moderate to severe language impairments but also suggest a specific link between ADHD and language impairment (Beitchman et al. 1986; Cantwell and Baker 1991; Cohen et al. 1993). Estimates of the overlap vary from 8% to 90%, depending on the precise definitions of each disorder, the methods used to diagnose them, and the nature of the communication problems (reviewed by Baker and Cantwell 1992; Tannock and Schachar 1996). One criticism levied at the prevalence estimates of language impairment in ADHD is that poor test performance may reflect problems in attention and behavior. The argument is that language tests implicate other cognitive abilities (e.g., attention, working memory, long-term memory) as well as receptive and expressive language. However, evidence that a substantial proportion of children with confirmed diagnosis of ADHD had test scores in the normal range mitigates this explanation (e.g., Oram et al. 1999).

Traditionally, two broad categories of communication disorders have been distinguished—*speech disorders* and *language disorders*, although more recently, another set of language-related problems have been recognized—*pragmatic language disorders*. Speech disorders refer to problems with the *motor production* of speech sounds (e.g., articulation, dysfluency that serves to interrupt the normal rhythm of speech, speech rate [too fast or too slow] that renders speech uninterpretable, and altered voice quality). In contrast, language disorders refer to problems with understanding and/or producing the conventional system of arbitrary signals and rules used for communication. Receptive language disorders may manifest as difficulties in understanding the meaning of words or sentence structure, following directions, and making inferences; typically, these difficulties also are accompanied by difficulties in expressive language. Expressive language disorders may be manifested by an extremely limited vocabulary, difficulties in word finding, use of immature or incorrect grammatical markers, difficulty with pronoun case marking or marking or maintaining tense, problems in ordering the words grammatically to convey a meaningful message, or omission of critical parts of sentences. By contrast, pragmatic language disorders are not language specific because they do not necessarily involve phonological, lexical, or syntactic problems. They refer to inappropriate use of language as a cognitive and social tool to convey information and to participate in the community and to learn. Pragmatic disorders may manifest as failure to understand or use social conventions, such as taking turns and other conversational rules, or failure to modulate tone, volume, or gestural accompaniments when expressing affect.

Speech Disorders in ADHD

In general, speech problems are less strongly related to ADHD than are language problems and, when they do exist, tend to co-occur with broader-band language problems (Beitchman et al. 1989; Cantwell and Baker 1991). On the other hand, some clinical and empirical reports indicated unmodulated volume, dysfluencies, and fast rate, suggesting some minor motor control problems in the speech of children with ADHD (Hamlett et al. 1987; Tannock et al. 1993; Zentall 1988).

Language Disorders in ADHD

A history of delayed onset of language, as assessed by the appearance of first words and short sentences, is more common in children with ADHD relative to their peers without ADHD. Delayed onset is reported in 6%–35% of children with ADHD compared with 2%–6% of non-ADHD children (Gross-Tsur et al. 1991; Hartsough and Lambert 1985; Ornoy et al. 1993; Szatmari et al. 1989). Findings apply to both DSM-IV ADHD and ICD-10 hyperkinetic disorder (e.g., Tripp et al. 1999).

The co-occurrence of receptive-expressive language impairments and ADHD symptoms emerges in the preschool years and continues through childhood into adolescence (e.g., Beitchman et al. 1987; Benasich et al. 1993; McGee et al. 1991; Ornoy et al. 1993). For example, Ornoy and colleagues (1993) found that 80% of the preschoolers who had the triad of language impairments, inattentiveness/hyperactivity, and soft neurological signs at age 3 years met the diagnosis for ADHD in middle childhood, and most had learning disabilities, particularly reading disorder. Community and clinical studies have documented language impairment in a substantial proportion (20%–60%) of school-age children with

ADHD (Beitchman et al. 1989; Cantwell and Baker 1991; Cohen et al. 1989; Oram et al. 1999; Tirosh and Cohen 1998).

Expressive language is particularly impaired (Baker and Cantwell 1992; Beitchman et al. 1987; Oram et al. 1999). Word retrieval problems and impairments in the basic language systems, such as phonology, semantics, and syntax, are seen (Cantwell and Baker 1991; Javorsky 1996; Oram et al. 1999; Purvis and Tannock 1997; Tannock et al. 1993). Word retrieval problems may be manifest by the use of nonspecific words (e.g., "that thing"), circumlocutions (e.g., "the thing you hit the um...nails with"), or reformulations (e.g., "the...um...thing—the water...uh...the puddle"). These difficulties are particularly apparent in situations that impose a continuous demand for specific vocabulary items and have time limitations, which are specified by the language test or activity or imposed by societal norms and expectations (e.g., when asked to name pictures on demand, retell stories, or describe past events). Impairments in expressive semantics, expressive syntax, and grammatical morphology are even more marked in those youngsters with concurrent phonological processing problems that underlie reading disorder (Javorsky 1996; Purvis and Tannock 1997). However, broad-based language impairment is evident in ADHD even in the presence of strong phonological skills.

Pragmatic Dysfunction in ADHD

Pragmatic deficits are highly associated with ADHD and occur even in those individuals with adequate phonological, morphological, syntactic, and semantic abilities (Humphries et al. 1994; Ludlow et al. 1978; Tannock and Schachar 1996). Moreover, they appear to be more strongly associated with ADHD than with learning disabilities (Humphries et al. 1994; Lapadat 1991). For example, Humphries and colleagues (1994) found that 60% of the boys with attention problems had pragmatic deficits, compared with 15% of those with learning disabilities and 7% of normally developing children. The high rate of pragmatic disorders in ADHD is not surprising because the defining features of ADHD include difficulties in the appropriate *timing* and *quantity* of language within social and learning contexts. For example, DSM-IV proposes that in social situations, 1) inattention may be expressed as frequent shifts in conversation, not listening to others, and not keeping one's mind on conversations; 2) hyperactivity may be manifested by excessive talkativeness; and 3) impulsivity may manifest itself as frequent and inappropriate initiation of conversation, excessive interruption of others, making comments out of turn, or blurting out answers before questions have been completed (American Psychiatric Association 1994, p. 79).

Pragmatic deficits associated with ADHD include 1) *excessive* verbal output during spontaneous conversations, during task transitions, and in play settings (Barkley et al. 1983; Zentall 1988); 2) *decreased* verbal output and more dysfluencies when confronted with tasks that require planning and organization of verbal responses, as in storytelling or when giving directions (Hamlett et al. 1987; Tannock et al. 1993; Zentall 1988); and 3) *timing problems* in terms of initiating conversation, taking turns, and maintaining or changing topics during conversation (Humphries et al. 1994; Zentall et al. 1983).

One important limitation of the existing research on communication skills in ADHD is that the studies have typically examined heterogeneous samples of children with ADHD and language impairment or ADHD but have not included a comparison group of children with language impairment alone. Thus, it is unclear which communication problems are uniquely associated with ADHD, with language impairment, or with the comorbid condition (Tannock and Schachar 1996).

Reading Disorders in ADHD

Developmental dyslexia, or reading disorder, refers to an unexpected difficulty in learning to read despite intact sensory and intellectual abilities and sufficient educational opportunities. Epidemiological and clinical studies suggest a comorbidity rate between ADHD and reading disorder of 15%–30% when relatively stringent criteria are used for defining each of the separate disorders (e.g., Semrud-Clikeman et al. 1992; Shaywitz et al. 1995). Investigators have proposed that learning disorders (including reading disorder) may be more commonly associated with inattention than with symptoms of hyperactivity-impulsivity (Barkley et al. 1990; Edelbrock et al. 1984; Hynd et al. 1991). Data from recent investigations of the DSM-IV subtypes of ADHD support this proposition to some extent. That is, academic underachievement and reading disorder are more common in the predominantly inattentive and combined types than in the hyperactive-impulsive type (e.g., Baumgaertel et al. 1995; Faraone et al. 1998; Gaub and Carlson 1997; Lamminmaki et al. 1995; Marshall et al. 1997; Paternite et al. 1996). These findings suggest a strong relation between reading disorder and inattention.

To achieve skill in reading, readers must gain access to the phonological units of language that writing systems represent. According to one model (Articulatory Phonology and Gestural Computational Model; Browman and Goldstein 1990, 1992; Browman et al. 1984; Liberman 1993; Saltzman and Munhall 1989), the grapheme-to-phoneme conversions require activation of motor-articulatory gestures. This model, which is an extension of older motor theories of speech perception (e.g., Liberman and Mattingly 1985), proposes that the basic phonological unit is the motor-articulatory gesture rather than mental representations, although this issue remains controversial.

The general consensus is that reading disorder stems from core deficits in the oral language skill of *phonemic awareness,* which refers to the ability to recognize and manipulate the phonemic constituents of speech (for reviews, see Adams 1990; Shaywitz et al. 1996; Vandervelden and Siegel 1996; Wagner et al. 1994; Wolf 1991). The motor-articulatory model may explain how phonological awareness develops and why it may be impaired in reading disorder (Heilman et al. 1996). Clearly, learning to read builds on the speech processes at many levels (Denckla 1993; Mann 1986), and language impairment is one of the most common precursors and correlates of reading disorder (e.g., Aram et al. 1984; Benasich et al. 1993; Bishop and Adams 1990).

Severe reading impairment is also characterized by deficits in *naming speed,* which involves the rapid oral production of the names of visually presented stimuli, such as colors, numbers, and digits (Denckla and Rudel 1976; Meyer et al. 1998; Wolf 1991).

Moreover, in languages with more transparent orthography (e.g., German, Spanish), poor readers continue to have slower reading rates and longer latencies on lexical retrieval tasks despite more rapid compensation for early phonological processing deficits (e.g., Wimmer 1993). According to one hypothesis, deficiencies in naming speed reflect inadequacies in a precise timing mechanism necessary to the development of orthographic codes and to their integration with phonological codes (Bowers and Wolf 1993). Naming speed is believed to be distinct from phonological processing, and individuals with both deficits are considered to have the most intractable form of dyslexia (Bowers 1995; Meyer et. al. 1998).

A third domain of impairment in reading disorder is in *motor coordination* (e.g., Denckla et al. 1985; Wolff et al. 1990). Children with reading disorder have difficulty maintaining the correct tempo, prosody, and rhythm in language, reading, and writing, as well as in other skilled manual actions (Denckla et al. 1985). Bimanual motor coordination and motor speech repetition are impaired in approximately 50% of individuals with reading disorder, ages 8–25 years (Wolff et al. 1990, 1995). Moreover, family studies of motor coordination and reading disorder suggest that reading impairment and motor coordination deficits cosegregate in approximately half of the affected relatives from families with reading disorder (Wolff et al. 1995). This constellation of impairments is physiologically plausible when viewed from the perspective of the Articulatory Phonology Model.

Phonological Processing and Naming Speed Deficits in ADHD

Most clinical studies that have controlled for comorbid reading disorder have found that both reading disorder and ADHD and reading disorder groups (classified on the basis of poor word identification skills) have deficits in phonological processing and naming speed but that ADHD and non-ADHD comparison groups do not (e.g., Ackerman and Dykman 1993, 1995; Felton and Wood 1989; Korkman and Pesonen 1994; Närhi and Ahonen 1995; Nigg et al. 1998; Pennington et al. 1993). Moreover, many studies that included measures of executive function or motor planning (which are believed to be central to ADHD) found impairments in those aspects of cognitive function in ADHD and ADHD and reading disorder groups but not in reading disorder or normal peer groups (Korkman and Pesonen 1994; Nigg et al. 1998). This pattern of findings suggests a double dissociation between ADHD and reading disorder in which reading disorder is associated with phonological processing and naming speed deficits, and ADHD is associated with executive function deficits. Also, these findings indicate that reading problems in children with ADHD and reading disorder cannot be attributed solely to the behavioral symptoms of ADHD.

In contrast, several recent studies have linked naming speed deficits to ADHD and other disorders (e.g., autism, spina bifida), thereby challenging the notion of the specificity to reading disorder (e.g., Brock and Knapp 1996; Carte et al. 1996; Dennis et al. 1999; Martinussen et al. 1998; Nigg et al. 1998; Piven and Palmer 1997; Schuerholz et al. 1995). One explanation of the discrepant findings relates to the different processing demands. Specifically, naming digits and letters can be automatized, whereas naming objects and colors is thought to require more controlled, effortful, semantic processing (Denckla and Rudel 1974, 1976; Wolf 1991). Naming speed deficits in ADHD generally have been found in the speed of naming colors and objects, consistent with the evidence of deficits in other tasks requiring controlled, effortful processing (e.g., Barkley et al. 1997; van der Meere 1996). Moreover, preliminary evidence suggests that slow naming in ADHD may not be caused by problems in naming ability per se (i.e., in rapid articulation of names) but by problems in pacing—that is, with the rapid recruitment of linguistic elements in ongoing speech. Specifically, during color naming, the interstimulus intervals between correctly named stimuli were longer and either were unfilled (i.e., silent) or contained extraneous elements such as stammering, fillers such as "um," and other dysfluencies (Bedard and Tannock 1999). Similar problems in rapid automatized naming have been observed in children with spina bifida, which is associated with congenital anomalies of the cerebellum (Dennis et al. 1999).

Additional Language and Motor Skill Deficits in ADHD and Reading Disorder

Children with ADHD and reading disorder are likely to have concomitant language impairments, including deficits in receptive and expressive abilities in semantic and syntactic components of language, as well as in narrative abilities (Purvis and Tannock 1997; Reader et al. 1994; Tannock et al. 1996). Also, several studies have documented controlled motor deficits in children with ADHD and reading disorder. For example, Denckla and colleagues (1985) reported that children with reading disorder and high levels of inattention and hyperactivity had more problems than those with reading disorder only in performing timed and repetitive motor tasks (e.g., "Time-to-Do 20," which included repetitive finger, arm, and leg movements). Also, preliminary evidence indicates that visuomotor problems may be more severe in ADHD and reading disorder than in either disorder alone (Närhi and Ahonen 1995). However, a recent controlled study concluded that deficits in timed motor movements were associated with ADHD per se, whereas naming speed deficits were associated with reading disorder, and that those with ADHD and reading disorder had impairments in both domains (Nigg et al. 1998).

Motor Impairments in ADHD

An association between motor coordination problems and ADHD has been documented in many epidemiological and clinical samples across different cultures. Moderate or severe motor problems among children with a primary diagnosis of ADHD have been reported, and, conversely, moderate or severe ADHD has been observed among children with a primary diagnosis of developmental coordination disorder (e.g., Carte et al. 1996; Denckla and Rudel 1978; I. C. Gillberg and Gillberg 1989; Kadesjo and Gillberg 1998, 1999; Mariani and Barkley 1997; Piek et al. 1999; Szatmari et al. 1989). The types of motor coordination problems reported are clinically significant and interfere with routine daily activities (e.g., fastening and unfastening clothes and shoes, schoolwork, play, sports) and are not attributable to chronological age, intellect, or other diagnosable neurological or psychiatric disorders (e.g., American Psychiatric Association 1994; World Health Organization 1992). These problems have been demonstrated with standardized tests of fine and gross motor skills as well as during neurological assessment for soft signs related to motor coordination and motor overflow movements (e.g., Carte et al. 1996; Kadesjo and Gillberg 1999; Mariani and Barkley 1997).

In samples of children with ADHD, prevalence estimates of motor problems vary from approximately 10% to 50% (e.g., Doyle et al. 1995; Hartsough and Lambert 1985; Piek et al. 1999). These motor coordination problems appear to be discernible in the preschool years (e.g., Mariani and Barkley 1997) and persist through the school-age years (e.g., Carte et al. 1996; Doyle et al. 1995; Hadders-Algra and Grooothuis 1999; Hellgren et al. 1993; Nigg et al. 1998; Whitmont and Clark 1996). Preliminary evidence suggests that the type and degree of motor difficulty may differ between DSM-IV subtypes of ADHD, with fine motor skills being more impaired in the inattentive subtype and gross motor skills more impaired in the combined type (Piek et al. 1999). Moreover, motor coordination problems may be more strongly related to inattention than to hyperactivity-impulsivity (Kadesjo and Gillberg 1998; Piek et al. 1999). Also, mild problems in the speed, rhythm, and precision of movement have been found to be more common in children with ADHD and comorbid reading disorder than in those with reading disorder alone (Denckla et al. 1985).

Conversely, a substantial proportion (50%–60%) of children with moderate or severe motor coordination problems (i.e., developmental coordination disorder) have ADHD or pronounced but subthreshold levels of ADHD symptoms (Kadesjo and Gillberg 1998, 1999; Landgren et al. 1996). Mild motor coordination problems (as reflected in the quality of general movements) are discernible in infancy, particularly between 2 and 4 months postterm (Hadders-Algra 1996; Prechtl et al. 1993). Normal general movements, which are complex movements involving the head, trunk, arms, and legs, are characterized by fluency, variation, and complexity (Prechtl 1990). In contrast, mildly abnormal general movements lack fluency and show problems in muscle coordination (Hadders-Algra et al. 1997). One study reported that mildly abnormal movements in early infancy predict mild neurological dysfunction (i.e., coordination problems) and ADHD at school age (Hadders-Algra and Groothuis 1999). Certainly, evidence indicates that developmental coordination disorder shows stability over time, at least in the school-age years (e.g., Kadesjo and Gillberg 1999).

Developmental coordination disorder, in turn, also is associated with speech and language impairments, visuoperceptual problems, and reading and spelling difficulties, as well as attention deficits (e.g., Fletcher-Flinn et al. 1997; Losse et al. 1991; Wilson and McKenzie 1998). For example, Whitmore and Bax (1990) reported that among a sample of children with deviant neurodevelopmental scores at age 5 years, 25% had learning disabilities at 2- to 5-year follow-up, compared with 4% with neurodevelopmental scores in the normal range. Also, children with either moderate or severe developmental coordination disorder had comorbid attentional, language, and reading problems (Kadesjo and Gillberg 1999).

Deficits in Attention, Motor Control, and Perception (DAMP)

The presenting behavioral symptoms of ADHD, the word identification problems in reading disorder, and the motor coordination problems in developmental coordination disorder are rarely isolated findings in each of these disorders. Rather, the complex pattern of impairments in attention/hyperactivity, language, reading, and motor coordination occurs frequently in each of the three clinical conditions that are currently differentiated by DSM-IV and ICD-10. By contrast, this common constellation of impairments is formally recognized in Nordic countries by the acronym DAMP (Kadesjo and Gillberg 1998; C. Gillberg et al. 1982).

DAMP is an umbrella term covering various combinations of deficits in attention, motor control, and perception in children with normal or low-normal intelligence and who do not meet the criteria for cerebral palsy (Rasmussen and Gillberg 1999). DAMP is conceptualized as a neurodevelopmental dysfunction syndrome, with a high degree of psychiatric comorbidity (e.g., Gillberg 1983; Hellgren et al. 1994). Accordingly, DAMP and ADHD overlap to a considerable extent: by definition, all children with severe DAMP meet criteria for ADHD, and, conversely, approximately 50% of the children with ADHD meet criteria for DAMP (Kadesjo and Gillberg 1999).

Longitudinal studies of well-defined subgroups from the general population in Sweden indicated that DAMP carries a worse prognosis than ADHD or developmental coordination disorder alone in terms of psychiatric, neurodevelopmental, and neurological problems at age 7 years, school problems at ages 10 and 13 years, and psychiatric and personality problems in adolescence (Gillberg 1983; I. C. Gillberg and Gillberg 1989; Hellgren et al. 1994; Rasmussen et al. 1983). Moreover, DAMP has been found to be more strongly associated with inattention than with hyperactivity-impulsivity and to be more strongly associated with classroom dysfunction than either ADHD or developmental coordination disorder alone (Kadesjo and Gillberg 1998).

Language problems occur in as many as 65% of children with DAMP (e.g., Landgren et al. 1998). The nature of these associated speech and language problems documented in Swedish samples of children with DAMP appears similar to that documented in North American samples of children with ADHD. For example, they include problems in articulation, stuttering, failure to adjust volume and pitch of voice to the context, as well as overall delay in language development in syntax, semantics, and pragmatics (Rasmussen and Gillberg 1999). Also, in a recent study of phonological working memory and speech discrimination, phonological working memory was impaired in the DAMP group but not in ADHD, and speech discrimination was unimpaired in both groups (Norrelgen et al. 1999).

No etiological explanations have been forwarded for this neurodevelopmental symptom complex, which is believed to have poorer prognosis than either of the single component conditions of ADHD and developmental coordination disorder (e.g., Hellgren et al. 1993, 1994; Kadesjo and Gillberg 1998; Landgren et al. 1996). However, a recent study implicated a range of nonoptimal familial, prenatal, and perinatal factors in the pathogenesis of DAMP (Landgren et al. 1998). For example, the following factors occurred at higher rates in children with DAMP compared with control subjects: lower socioeconomic class, familial language disorder or learning disorders and familial motor clumsiness, maternal smoking during pregnancy, language problems in preschool years, sleep problems (nighttime snoring), and gastrointestinal disorders (Landgren et al. 1998).

Stimulant Effects on Language, Reading, and Motor Control Problems in ADHD

Few controlled investigations of the effect of stimulant medication on problems in oral language, basic processes involved in reading, and motor coordination that frequently coexist with ADHD have been done, and the limited data available are disappointing. Few systematic effects have been found on language or reading (Tannock 1999). The few discernible effects on language appear to be restricted to the quality or style of the children's language in that it appears less vigorous and intense (e.g., Whalen et al. 1979). Also, stimulant medication may increase self-monitoring and correction, but it does not appear to have any effect on the basic subsystems of language (phonology, syntax, semantics) or on the effectiveness, functional content, or dysfluency of children's communication (Hamlett et al. 1987; Tannock 1999; Whalen et al. 1979). However, given the strong evidence that methylphenidate use results in reduced parent and teacher ratings of hyperactivity (e.g., talkativeness) and impulsivity (e.g., talking out of turn, blurting out), one effect of stimulant medication may be to improve the timing of spoken language. This effect has not been investigated systematically.

In contrast to the incontrovertible evidence of stimulant effects on academic productivity (i.e., quantity of assigned work completed), little evidence indicates that stimulants have any immediate effect on phonological processing, the speed or accuracy of reading, or reading comprehension per se (Ballinger et al. 1984; Balthazor et al. 1991; Forness et al. 1992; Richardson et al. 1988). Moreover, the effect of stimulant medication on reading comprehension itself (as opposed to productivity measures) is unclear, primarily because of the lack of data (Ballinger et al. 1984; Brock and Knapp 1996; Cherkes-Julkowski et al. 1995). However, some evidence suggests that stimulant medication may enhance verbal retrieval mechanisms involved in word recognition (Ballinger et al. 1984; Evans et al. 1986; Peeke et al. 1984; Richardson et al. 1988). Also, several recent controlled studies suggested that methylphenidate may enhance naming speed and accuracy of contingency naming (Douglas et al. 1995; Martinussen et al. 1998).

Although stimulant medication has been observed to improve handwriting and some aspects of motor sequencing and fine motor coordination in children with ADHD (Lerer and Lerer 1976; Lerer et al. 1977), effects on other fine motor skills, gross motor skills, or motor coordination are not observed routinely. By contrast, one consistent finding is of decreased variability in response latencies that is sometimes accompanied by overall speeding of responses.

In summary, little credible evidence exists to date that stimulant medication has systematic and robust effects on the type of language, reading, or motor skill problems that frequently accompany ADHD. No study to date has examined stimulant effects in ADHD groups with and without the combination of problems (i.e., inattention/hyperactivity, language, reading, motor coordination). Thus, it is not possible to determine whether this constellation of problems alters the typical treatment response in ADHD alone.

Cerebellar Dysfunction as a Common Etiology in ADHD, Reading Disorder, and Developmental Coordination Disorder

In ADHD research, several explanations have been proposed for the comorbidity with reading disorder and with language impairment. For example, ADHD and reading disorder are generally considered etiologically distinct disorders, although a shared genetic etiology has been speculated for some cases (e.g., Faraone et al. 1993; Gilger et al. 1992; Shaywitz and Shaywitz 1991). Candidate explanations for the frequent association of psychiatric disorder (particularly ADHD) and general linguistic impairment include a common etiological factor, such as "neurodevelopmental immaturity" (Beitchman et al. 1989) or a deficiency in processing rapidly changing stimuli, particularly across modalities (Tallal et al. 1989), and shared genetic influences (Stevenson et al. 1993). The latter explanation was offered to account for the frequent overlap of ADHD and spelling disability, each of which demonstrates substantial heritability (DeFries et al. 1991; Gillis et al. 1992). More recently, Stevenson (1996) presented a hypothetical account of the developmental changes in disorders of language, reading, and behavior (internalizing and externalizing) and in their interrelationships: genetic factors were implicated.

The complex pattern of concurrent impairments in language, reading, and motor coordination (in particular) has barely been recognized in ADHD research. These additional problems are generally conceptualized as comorbidities that have no synergistic effect on ADHD (e.g., Jensen et al. 1997). However, Barkley et al. (1997) proposed that impairments in language (e.g., verbal working memory, verbal fluency) and motor control (e.g., execution of novel/complex motor sequences) are integral to ADHD because of their dependency on behavioral inhibition, which is conceptualized as the fundamental deficit in ADHD.

Alternatively, cerebellar dysfunction may provide a "unified account" of the complex pattern of impairments in language, reading, motor coordination, and inattention/hyperactivity, which is not specific to ADHD (or to reading disorder or developmental coordination disorder), but which represents an important behavioral phenotype. This proposition is based on three outcomes of research: 1) current understanding of the role of the cerebellum; 2) evidence of cerebellar dysfunction in reading disorder; and 3) evidence of cerebellar dysfunction in ADHD.

Cerebellar Role in Motor Control, Timing, and Cognition

Strong and consistent evidence (across animal studies and clinical and neuroimaging studies in humans) shows that the cerebellum plays an important role in motor control, including the regulation of balance, posture and gait, fine motor control, acquisition and automatization of skilled voluntary movement, and classical condition of motor responses (e.g., Daum and Ackerman 1995; Ghez 1991; Ito 1993). The cerebellum is essential for the quality of movement: cerebellar lesions impair the quality of movement (e.g., fluency) but do not abolish movement (Gilman 1994).

Some have proposed that the cerebellum is one component in a cognitive timing system that contributes to the control of movement and also to performance on nonmotor tasks—perceptual tasks—that require the precise representation of temporal information (Daum and Ackerman 1995; Ivry 1997). The precise representation of temporal information is required to be able to predict and anticipate impending events, as well as to organize and plan sequences of action. For example, the preparation of fast responses benefits from the ability to predict precisely the point in time when an impending event requires a response. Temporal processing (time perception) is a complex cognitive activity, comprising multiple component processes that engage multiple brain regions, including the basal ganglia, prefrontal cortex, and neocerebellum (Gibbon et al. 1997; Harrington et al. 1998; Ivry and Hazeltine 1995; Mangels et al. 1998).

Lesion studies have provided evidence for the role of the cerebellum in timing (Ivry and Keele 1989; Jueptner et al. 1995; Mangels et al. 1998; Maquet et al. 1996; Nicolson et al. 1999). For example, patients with cerebellar lesions showed poor acuity on perceptual tasks that require precise timing, such as duration discrimination or velocity discrimination (Ivry and Keele 1989). Because these patients did not show perceptual deficits on nontemporal tasks, such as loudness or pitch discrimination, the cerebellum appears to contribute to those tasks that require a precise representation of fine timing between sensory and motor events (Casini and Ivry 1999; Ivry 1997). Also, positron-emission tomography (PET) studies provided more direct evidence of cerebellar involvement in time perception (Jupetner et al. 1995; Maquet et al. 1996). Findings from these studies suggest that the cerebellum is essential for providing an accurate representation of temporal information, whereas the prefrontal cortex subserves supportive functions associated with the acquisition, maintenance, monitoring, and organization of temporal representations in working memory (Casini and Ivry 1999; Ivry 1997; Mangels et al. 1998).

More recently, the cerebellum has been implicated in higher-order cognitive functioning and nonmotor learning, including visuospatial abilities, verbal fluency, language processing, and categorical speech perception (Ackerman et al. 1997; Akshoomoff and Courchesne 1992; Fiez et al. 1992; Schmahmann and Sherman 1998; Thach 1997). This issue remains under debate (Daum and Ackerman 1995; Ivry 1997).

Cerebellar Dysfunction in Reading Disorder

In reading disorder research, the observed overlap between impairments in motor coordination and perceptual and phonological skills (and spelling problems) has been attributed to mild cerebellar dysfunction (e.g., Denckla 1993; Nicolson and Fawcett 1994a; Nicolson et al. 1995, 1999; Rae et al. 1998; Wolff et al. 1990). For example, behavioral studies have found that children with reading disorder have impairments on classic clinical tests of cerebellar function (e.g., Nicolson and Fawcett 1994b). In a recent study, 80% of a sample of 60 children with reading disorder showed behavioral signs of cerebellar deficits (Nicolson et al. 1999). Also, a theoretical study found impaired time estimation in children with reading disorder but no impairment in the control task of loudness estimation (Nicolson et al. 1995) when methods known to require cerebellar activity were used (Ivry and Keele 1989; Jueptner et al. 1995; Mangels et al. 1998).

Direct evidence of cerebellar dysfunction during motor tasks is provided by a recent PET study of brain activation in adults with dyslexia as they either performed a prelearned sequence of finger movements or learned a novel sequence (Nicolson et al. 1999). Abnormalities in cerebellar activation in the adults with dyslexia were reflected by significantly lower activation levels in the right cerebellar cortex and left cingulate gyrus when executing the prelearned sequence and in the right cerebellar cortex when learning the new sequence. These findings provide direct evidence that the behavioral signs of motor impairments reflect underlying abnormalities in activation of the right cerebellar cortex (Nicolson et al. 1999; Rae et al. 1998) as well as in the left temporoparietal cortex (Rae et al. 1998). These cerebellar findings can be readily integrated with the proposed impairment of magnocellular development

(Livingstone et al. 1991; J. Stein et al. 1997). As explained by Rae and colleagues (1998), this is because one major output of the visual magnocellular system projects to the posterior parietal cortex, and the largest output of the posterior parietal cortex projects to the contralateral cerebellar hemisphere (Stein and Glickstein 1992).

Finally, family studies of pedigrees with dyslexia suggest that impairments in temporal resolution in motor action may constitute a behavioral phenotype transmitted in familial dyslexia (Wolff et al. 1995, 1996). However, the coexistence of impairments in attention/hyperactivity is rarely considered in current investigations of reading disorder (with the notable exception of Nicolson et al. 1999).

Cerebellar Dysfunction in ADHD

Findings from behavioral, cognitive, and neuroimaging studies provide converging evidence of cerebellar dysfunction in ADHD. As discussed earlier in this chapter, numerous behavioral studies have identified deficits in children with ADHD on clinical tests of cerebellar function, including problems in the timing, precision, fine and gross motor skills, balance, rhythmicity, and sequenced movements (e.g., Denckla and Rudel 1976; Nigg et al. 1998; Piek et al. 1999). Also, several studies have reported time perception impairments in children with ADHD (Barkley et al. 1997; Capella et al. 1997; Rubia et al. 1999; Tannock 1999). For example, one study investigated time perception in children with ADHD, children with ADHD and reading disorder, and a comparison group with psychophysical methods similar to those of Ivry (e.g., Ivry and Keele 1989). Tasks included duration discrimination (target duration of 400 ms vs. a foil duration), frequency discrimination (a control task to evaluate general perceptual ability), and duration estimation using the method of reproduction for intervals of 400 ms, 2,000 ms, and 6,000 ms. Both ADHD groups were impaired in duration estimation and in duration discrimination but not in frequency discrimination, consistent with cerebellar dysfunction (Tannock 1999).

More direct evidence of cerebellar anomalies in ADHD is provided by neuroimaging studies. For example, recent magnetic resonance imaging studies of cerebellar structure in ADHD documented a reduction in cerebellar volume (Castellanos et al. 1996), specifically in the volume of the inferior posterior vermis (lobules VIII–X), with sparing of the superior posterior lobes (lobules VI/ VII). These differences remained robust even after adjustment for overall brain volume (Berquin et al. 1998; Mostofsky et al. 1998). Notably, the inferior cerebellar vermis has been shown to play a role in time perception, along with other brain regions, prefrontal cortex, and cingulate cortex (Jueptner et al. 1995). Importantly, a review of neuroimaging studies of ADHD reveals evidence of subtle changes in brain morphology (typically reduced regional volumes or altered asymmetries) in those brain regions required for the efficient timing of sequential movements, including the cerebellum, that play a unique role in representing temporal information (Tannock 1998).

The cerebellum is one of the first brain regions to be differentiated and has a prolonged cycle of maturation, as reflected by patterns of myelination. Thus, its early development may be altered by genetic mechanisms and/or by nonoptimal environmental events in early postnatal development. The preceding review suggests that subgroups of individuals within many of the developmental disorders currently differentiated by DSM-IV (ADHD, reading disorder, language impairment, developmental coordination disorder) have the complex constellation of impairments of inattention/hyperactivity, speech and language problems, reading difficulties, and motor control problems. Moreover, cerebellar dysfunction is evident in ADHD and reading disorder (and in developmental coordination disorder by extrapolation). Could this be a possible explanation of this constellation of developmental impairments? This exposition should not be interpreted as a "cerebellar" hypothesis of ADHD. Rather, it is proposed that this constellation of problems may reflect a behavioral phenotype that is not specific to ADHD or to any specific disorder currently differentiated by DSM-IV but that may be transmitted in families.

Clinical Implications

Irrespective of possible mechanisms or etiology, this review has provided evidence that individuals with ADHD frequently have concurrent impairments in language, reading, and motor coordination; that individuals with reading disorder frequently have language impairments and motor coordination problems; and that children with developmental coordination disorder frequently have problems in language, reading, and inattention/hyperactivity. Previous research has shown that concurrent communication disorders in ADHD often are undetected unless a systematic language assessment is included in the assessment for ADHD (Cohen et al. 1989, 1993). This likely holds true for motor coordination (and reading, but to a lesser extent because teachers are sensitive to reading skills). Accordingly, findings from the present review highlight the importance of including an evaluation of language, reading, and motor skills and inattention/hyperactivity routinely in the assessment of children referred to specialty clinics (e.g., learning disabilities, ADHD), neurology, developmental pediatrics, psychiatry, and so on.

The occurrence of this constellation of symptoms also poses challenges for treatment. Little evidence to date indicates that stimulant treatment for ADHD will have any systematic or substantive effect on concurrent language, reading, or motor problems. Second, the presence of concurrent problems in language and motor coordination may preclude any benefits typically accrued from behavior therapies that rely on verbal mediation (e.g., cognitive-behavior therapy), or from specific remediation programs for reading that place heavy demands on writing and oral language. From the child's perspective, however, problems arising from not being able to read, understand peer language, or catch a ball, and the resultant effect on friendships, may be far more impairing than the behavioral symptoms of ADHD that may have motivated the referral.

References

Ackerman H, Graber S, Hertrich I, et al: Categorical speech perception in cerebellar disorders. Brain Lang 60:323–331, 1997
Ackerman PT, Dykman RA: Phonological processes, confrontational naming, and immediate memory in dyslexia. J Learn Disabil 26:597–609, 1993

Ackerman PT, Dykman RA: Reading-disabled students with and without comorbid arithmetic disability. Developmental Neuropsychology 11:151–371, 1995

Adams MJ: Beginning to Read: Thinking and Learning About Print. Cambridge, MA, MIT Press, 1990

Akshoomkoff NA, Courchesne E: A new role for the cerebellum in cognitive operations. Behav Neurosci 106:731–738, 1992

American Psychiatric Association: Diagnostic and Statistical Manual of Mental Disorders, 4th Edition. Washington, DC, American Psychiatric Association, 1994

Aram DM, Ekelman B, Nation JE: Preschoolers with language disorders: 10 years later. Journal of Speech and Hearing Research 27:232–244, 1984

Baker L, Cantwell DP: Attention deficit disorder and speech/language disorders. Comprehensive Mental Health Care 2:3–16, 1992

Ballinger CT, Varley CK, Nolen PA: Effects of methylphenidate on reading in children with attention deficit disorder. Am J Psychiatry 141:1590–1593, 1984

Balthazor MJ, Wagner RK, Pelham WE: The specificity of effects of stimulant medication on classroom learning-related measures of cognitive processing for attention deficit disorder children. J Abnorm Child Psychol 19:35–52, 1991

Barkley RA: Attention-Deficit Hyperactivity Disorder: A Handbook for Diagnosis and Treatment. New York, Guilford, 1998

Barkley RA, Cunningham CE, Karlsson J: The speech of hyperactive children and their mothers: comparison with normal children and stimulant drug effects. J Learn Disabil 16:105–110, 1983

Barkley RA, Fischer M, Edelbrock CS, et al: The adolescent outcome of hyperactive children diagnosed by research criteria, I: an 8-year prospective follow-up study. J Am Acad Child Adolesc Psychiatry 29:546–557, 1990

Barkley RA, Koplowicz S, Anderson T, et al: Sense of time in children with ADHD: effects of duration, distraction, and stimulant medication. Journal of the International Neuropsychological Society 3:359–369, 1997

Baumgaertel A, Wolraich ML, Dietrich M: Comparison of diagnostic criteria for attention deficit disorders in a German elementary school sample. J Am Acad Child Adolesc Psychiatry 34:629–638, 1995

Bedard AC, Tannock R: Naming speed and stimulant effects in children with ADHD. Poster presented at the Samual Lunenfeld Summer Student Symposium, The Hospital for Sick Children, Toronto, Ontario, Canada, July 28, 1999

Beitchman JH, Nair R, Clegg M, et al: Prevalence of psychiatric disorders in children with speech and language disorders. J Am Acad Child Psychiatry 25:528–535, 1986

Beitchman J, Tuckett M, Batth S: Language delay and hyperactivity in preschoolers: evidence for a distinct group of hyperactives. Can J Psychiatry 32:683–687, 1987

Beitchman JH, Hood J, Rochon J, et al: Empirical classification of speech/language impairment in children, II: behavioral characteristics. J Am Acad Child Adolesc Psychiatry 28:118–123, 1989

Benasich AA, Curtiss S, Tallal P: Language, learning, and behavioral disturbances in childhood: a longitudinal perspective. J Am Acad Child Adolesc Psychiatry 32:585–594, 1993

Berquin PC, Giedd JN, Jacobsen LK, et al: Cerebellum in attention-deficit hyperactivity disorder: a morphometric MRI study. Neurology 50:1087–1093, 1998

Biederman J, Newcorn J, Sprich S: Comorbidity of attention deficit hyperactivity disorder with conduct, depressive, anxiety and other disorders. Am J Psychiatry 148:564–577, 1991

Bird H, Canino G, Rubio-Stipec M, et al: Estimates of the presence of childhood maladjustment in a community survey in Puerto Rico. Arch Gen Psychiatry 45:1120–1126, 1988

Bishop DVM: The underlying nature of specific language impairment. J Child Psychol Psychiatry 33:3–66, 1992

Bishop DVM, Adams C: A prospective study of the relationship between specific language impairment, phonological disorders and reading retardation. J Child Psychol Psychiatry 31:1027–1050, 1990

Bishop DV, North T, Donlan C: Genetic basis of specific language impairment: evidence from a twin study. Dev Med Child Neurol 37:56–71, 1995

Bowers PG: Tracing symbol naming speed's unique contribution to reading disabilities over time. Reading and Writing: An Interdisciplinary Journal 7:189–216, 1995

Bowers PG, Wolf M: Theoretical links among naming speed, precise timing mechanisms and orthographic skills in dyslexia. Reading and Writing: An Interdisciplinary Journal 5:69–85, 1993

Brock SE, Knapp PK: Reading comprehension abilities of children with attention-deficit/hyperactivity disorder. Journal of Attention Disorders 1:173–185, 1996

Browman CP, Goldstein L: Gestural specification using dynamically-defined articulatory gestures. Journal of Phonetics 18:411–424, 1990

Browman CP, Goldstein L: Articulatory phonology: an overview. Phonetica 49:155–180, 1992

Browman CP, Golstein L, Kelso JAS, et al: Articulatory synthesis from underlying dynamics. J Acoust Soc Am 75:S22–S23, 1984

Bruck M: Persistence of dyslexics' phonological awareness deficits. Dev Psychol 28:874–886, 1992

Cantwell DP, Baker L: Prevalence and type of psychiatric disorder and developmental disorders in three speech and language groups. J Commun Disord 20:151–160, 1987

Cantwell DP, Baker L: Psychiatric and Developmental Disorders in Children With Communication Disorder. Washington, DC, American Psychiatric Press, 1991

Capella B, Gentile JR, Juliano DB: Time estimation by hyperactive and normal children. Percept Mot Skills 44:787–790, 1997

Cardon LR, DeFries JC, Filker DW, et al: Quantitative trait locus for reading disability on chromosome 6. Science 266:276–279, 1994

Caron C, Rutter M: Comorbidity in child psychopathology: concepts, issues and research strategies. J Child Psychol Psychiatry 32:1063–1080, 1991

Carte ET, Nigg JT, Hinshaw SP: Neuropsychological functioning, motor speed, and language processing in boys with and without ADHD. J Abnorm Child Psychol 24:481–498, 1996

Casini L, Ivry RB: Effects of divided attention on temporal processing in patients with lesions of the cerebellum or frontal lobe. Neuropsychology 13:10–21, 1999

Caspi A, Moffitt TE, Newman DL, et al: Behavioral observations at age 3 years predict adult psychiatric disorders: longitudinal evidence from a birth cohort. Arch Gen Psychiatry 53:1033–1039, 1996

Castellanos FX, Giedd JN, Marsh WL, et al: Quantitative brain magnetic resonance imaging in attention-deficit hyperactivity disorder. Arch Gen Psychiatry 53:607–616, 1996

Cherkes-Julkowski M, Stolzenberg J, Hatzes N, et al: Methodological issues in assessing the relationships among ADD, medication effects and reading performance. Learning Disabilities: A Multidisciplinary Journal 6:21–30, 1995

Clements SD: Task Force One: Minimal Brain Dysfunction in Children (National Institute of Neurological Diseases and Blindness, Monograph No 3). Rockville, MD, U.S. Department of Health, Education and Welfare, 1966

Cohen NJ, Davine M, Meloche-Kelly M: Prevalence of unsuspected language disorders in a child psychiatric population. J Am Acad Child Adolesc Psychiatry 28:107–111, 1989

Cohen N, Davine M, Horodezky N, et al: Unsuspected language impairment in psychiatrically disturbed children: prevalence and language and behavioral characteristics. J Am Acad Child Adolesc Psychiatry 32:595–603, 1993

Cook EH, Stein MA, Krasowski MD, et al: Association of attention-deficit disorder and the dopamine transporter gene. Am J Hum Genet 56:993–998, 1995

Daum I, Ackerman H: Cerebellar contributions to cognition. Behavioral Brain Research 67:201–210, 1995

DeFries JC, Stevenson J, Gillis JJ, et al: Genetic etiology of spelling deficits in the Colorado and London twin studies of reading disability. Reading and Writing 3:271–283, 1991

Denckla MB: A neurologist's overview of developmental dyslexia. Ann N Y Acad Sci 682:23–26, 1993

Denckla MB, Rudel RG: "Rapid automatized naming" of pictured objects, colors, letters, and numbers by normal children. Cortex 10:186–202, 1974

Denckla MB, Rudel RG: Rapid "automatized" naming (RAN): dyslexia differentiated from other learning disabilities. Neuropsychologia 14:471–479, 1976

Denckla MB, Rudel RG: Anomalies of motor development in hyperactive boys. Ann Neurol 3:231–233, 1978

Denckla MB, Rudel RG, Chapman C, et al: Motor proficiency in dyslexic children with and without attentional disorders. Arch Neurol 42:228–231, 1985

Dennis M, Hetherington CR, Spiegler BJ, et al: Functional consequences of congenital cerebellar dysmorphologies and acquired cerebellar lesions of childhood, in The Changing Nervous System: Neurobehavioral Consequences of Early Brain Disorders. Edited by Broman SH, Fletcher JM. New York, Oxford University Press, 1999, pp 172–198

Douglas VI, Barr RG, Desilets J, et al: Do high doses of stimulants impair flexible thinking in attention-deficit hyperactivity disorder? J Am Acad Child Adolesc Psychiatry 34:877–885, 1995

Doyle S, Wallen M, Whitmont S: Motor skills in Australian children with attention deficit hyperactivity disorder. Occupational Therapy International 2:229–240, 1995

Edelbrock C, Costello AJ, Kessler MD: Empirical corroboration of attention deficit disorder. J Am Acad Child Adolesc Psychiatry 23:285–290, 1984

Evans RW, Gualtieri CT, Amara I: Methylphenidate and memory: dissociated effects in hyperactive children. Psychopharmacology 90:211–216, 1986

Faraone SV, Biederman J, Lehman BK, et al: Evidence for the independent familial transmission of attention deficit hyperactivity disorder and learning disabilities: results from a family genetic study. Am J Psychiatry 150:891–895, 1993

Faraone SV, Biederman J, Weber W, et al: Psychiatric, neuropsychological, and psychosocial features of DSM-IV subtypes of attention-deficit/hyperactivity disorder: results from a clinically referred sample. J Am Acad Child Adolesc Psychiatry 37:185–193, 1998

Federal Register. Washington, DC, National Archives and Records Administration, 1990

Felton RH, Wood FB: Cognitive deficits in reading disability and attention deficit disorder. J Learn Disabil 22:3–13, 1989

Fiez JA, Petersen SE, Cheny MK, et al: Impaired non-motor learning and error detection associated with cerebellar damage. Brain 115:155–178, 1992

Fletcher-Flinn CM, Elmes H, Strugnell D: Visual perception and phonological factors in the acquisition of literacy among children with congenital developmental coordination disorder. Dev Med Child Neurol 39:158–166, 1997

Forness SR, Swanson JM, Cantwell DP, et al: Stimulant medication and reading performance: follow-up on sustained dose in ADHD boys with and without conduct disorders. J Learn Disabil 25:115–123, 1992

Gaub M, Carlson CL: Behavioral characteristics of DSM-IV subtypes in a school-based population. J Abnorm Child Psychol 25:103–111, 1997

Ghez C: The cerebellum, in Principles of Neural Science, 3rd Edition. Edited by Kandel ER, Schwartz JH, Jessell TM. New York, Elsevier Science, 1991, pp 626–646

Gibbon J, Malapani CL, Dale CL, et al: Toward a neurobiology of temporal cognition: advances and challenges. Curr Opin Neurobiol 7:170–184, 1997

Gilger JW, Pennington BF, DeFries C: A twin study of the etiology of comorbidity: attention deficit hyperactivity disorder and dyslexia. J Am Acad Child Adolesc Psychiatry 31:343–348, 1992

Gillberg C: Perceptual, motor and attentional deficits in Swedish primary school children: some child psychiatric aspects. J Child Psychol Psychiatry 24:377–403, 1983

Gillberg C, Rasmussen P, Carlstrom G, et al: Perceptual, motor and attentional deficits in six-year-old children: epidemiological aspects. J Child Psychol Psychiatry 23:131–144, 1982

Gillberg IC, Gillberg C: Children with preschool minor neurodevelopmental disorders, IV: behaviour and school achievement at age 13. Dev Med Child Neurol 31:3–13, 1989

Gillis JJ, Gilger JW, Pennington BF, et al: Attention deficit hyperactivity disorder in reading disabled twins: evidence for a genetic etiology. J Abnorm Child Psychol 20:303–315, 1992

Gilman S: Cerebellar control of movement. Ann Neurol 35:3–4, 1994

Grigorenko EL, Wood FB, Meyer MS, et al: Susceptibility loci for distinct components of developmental dyslexia on chromosomes 6 and 15. Am J Hum Genet 60:27–39, 1997

Gross-Tsur V, Shalev RS, Amir N: Attention deficit disorder: association with familial-genetic factors. Pediatr Neurol 7:258–261, 1991

Gualtieri CT, Koriath U, Van Bourgondien M, et al: Language disorders in children referred for psychiatric services. J Am Acad Child Psychiatry 22:165–171, 1983

Hadders-Algra M: Assessment of general movements: a valuable technique for detecting brain dysfunction in young infants. Acta Paediatr 416 (suppl):39–43, 1996

Hadders-Algra M, Groothuis AMC: Quality of general movements in infancy is related to neurological dysfunction, ADHD, and aggressive behaviour. Dev Med Child Neurol 41:381–391, 1999

Hadders-Algra M, Klip-Van den Nieuwendijk AWJ, Martijn A, et al: Assessment of general movements: towards a better understanding of a sensitive method to evaluate brain functioning in young infants. Dev Med Child Neurol 39:88–98, 1997

Hamlett KW, Pellegrini DS, Conners CK: An investigation of executive processes in the problem-solving of attention deficit disorder-hyperactive children. J Pediatr Psychol 12:227–240, 1987

Harrington DL, Haaland KY, Knight RT: Cortical networks underlying mechanisms of time perception. J Neurosci 18:1085–1095, 1998

Hartsough CS, Lambert NM: Medical factors in hyperactive and normal children: prenatal, developmental, and health history findings. Am J Orthopsychiatry 55:190–201, 1985

Heilman KM, Voeller K, Alexander AW: Developmental dyslexia: a motor-articulatory feedback hypothesis. Ann Neurol 39:407–412, 1996

Hellgren L, Gillberg C, Gillberg IC, et al: Children with deficits in attention, motor control and perception (DAMP) almost grown up: general health at 16 years. Dev Med Child Neurol 35:881–892, 1993

Hellgren L, Gillberg IC, Bagenholm A, et al: Children with deficits in attention, motor control and perception (DAMP) almost grown up: psychiatric and personality disorders at age 16 years. J Child Psychol Psychiatry 35:1255–1271, 1994

Hinshaw SP: Externalizing behavior problems and academic underachievement in childhood and adolescence: causal relationships and underlying mechanisms. Psychol Bull 111:127–155, 1992

Humphries T, Koltun H, Malone M, et al: Teacher-identified oral language difficulties among boys with attention problems. Developmental and Behavioral Pediatrics 15:92–98, 1994

Hynd GW, Lorys AR, Semrud-Clikeman M, et al: Attention deficit disorder without hyperactivity: a distinct behavioral and neurocognitive syndrome. J Child Neurol 6 (suppl):S37–S43, 1991

Ito M: Movement and thought: identical control mechanisms by the cerebellum. Trends Neurosci 16:448–450, 1993

Ivry R: Cerebellar timing systems. Int Rev Neurobiol 41:555–573, 1997

Ivry RB, Hazeltine RE: Perception and production of temporal intervals across a range of durations: evidence for a common timing mechanism. J Exp Psychol Hum Percept Perform 21:3–18, 1995

Ivry RB, Keele SW: Timing functions of the cerebellum. J Cogn Neurosci 1:136–152, 1989

Javorsky J: An examination of youth with attention-deficit/hyperactivity disorder and language learning disabilities: a clinical study. J Learn Disabil 29:247–258, 1996

Jensen PS, Martin D, Cantwell DP: Comorbidity in ADHD: implications for research, practice, and DSM-V. J Am Acad Child Adolesc Psychiatry 36:1065–1079, 1997

Jueptner M, Rijntjes M, Weiller C, et al: Localization of a cerebellar timing process using PET. Neurology 45:1540–1545, 1995

Kadesjo B, Gillberg C: Attention deficits and clumsiness in Swedish 7-year-old children. Dev Med Child Neurol 40:796–804, 1998

Kadesjo B, Gillberg C: Developmental coordination disorder in Swedish 7-year-old children. J Am Acad Child Adolesc Psychiatry 38:820–828, 1999

Kalverboer AF: Neurobehavioural relationships in children: new facts, new fictions. Early Hum Dev 34:169–177, 1993

Korkman M, Pesonen AE: A comparison of neuropsychological test profiles of children with attention deficit-hyperactivity disorder and/or learning disability. J Learn Disabil 27:383–392, 1994

LaHoste GJ, Swanson JM, Wigal SB, et al: Dopamine D4 receptor gene polymorphism is associated with attention deficit hyperactivity disorder. Mol Psychiatry 1:121–124, 1996

Lamminmaki T, Ahonen T, Narhi V, et al: Attention deficit hyperactivity disorder subtypes: are there differences in academic problems? Developmental Neuropsychology 11:297–310, 1995

Landgren M, Pettersson R, Kjellman B, et al: ADHD, DAMP and other neurodevelopmental/psychiatric disorders in 6-year-old children: epidemiology and co-morbidity. Dev Med Child Neurol 38:891–906, 1996

Landgren M, Kjellman B, Gillberg C: Attention deficit disorder with developmental coordination disorders. Archives of Diseases of Childhood 79:207–212, 1998

Lapadat JC: Pragmatic language skills of students with language and/or learning disabilities: a quantitative synthesis. J Learn Disabil 24:147–158, 1991

Lerer RJ, Lerer P: The effects of methylphenidate on the soft neurological signs of hyperactive children. Pediatrics 57:521–525, 1976

Lerer RJ, Lerer P, Artner J: The effects of methylphenidate on the handwriting of children with minimal brain dysfunction. J Pediatr 91:127–132, 1977

Lewis C, Hitch GJ, Walker P: The prevalence of specific arithmetic difficulties and specific reading difficulties in 9- to 10-year-old boys and girls. J Child Psychol Psychiatry 35:283–292, 1994

Liberman AM: In speech perception, time is not what it seems. Ann N Y Acad Sci 682:264–271, 1993

Liberman AM, Mattingly IG: The motor theory of speech perception revised. Cognition 21:1–36, 1985

Livingstone MS, Rosen GD, Drislane FW, et al: Physiological and anatomical evidence for a magnocellular deficit in developmental dyslexia. Proc Natl Acad Sci U S A 88:7943–7947, 1991

Losse A, Henderson SE, Elliman D, et al: Clumsiness in children—do they grow out of it? a 10-year follow-up study. Dev Med Child Neurol 33:55–68, 1991

Ludlow C, Rapoport J, Basich C, et al: Differential effects of dextroamphetamine on language performance in hyperactive and normal boys, in Treatment of Hyperactive and Learning Disordered Children. Edited by Knights R, Bakker D. Baltimore, MD, University Park Press, 1978, pp 185–205

Ludlow CL, Cudahy EA, Bassich C, et al: Auditory processing skills of hyperactive, language impaired and reading disabled boys, in Central Auditory Processing Disorders: Problems of Speech, Language, and Learning. Edited by Lasky EZ, Katz, J. Baltimore, MD, University Park Press, 1983, pp 163–184

Mangels JA, Ivry RB, Shimizu N: Dissociable contributions of the prefrontal and neocerebellar cortex to time perception. Cognitive Brain Research 7:15–39, 1998

Mann VA: Why some children encounter reading problems: the contribution of difficulties with language processing and phonological sophistication to early reading disability, in Psychological and Educational Perspectives on Learning Disabilities. Edited by Torggeson JK, Wong BYL. New York, Academic, 1986, pp 133–149

Maquet P, Lejeune H, Pouthas V, et al: Brain activation induced by estimation of duration: a PET study. Neuroimage 3:119–126, 1996

Mariani MA, Barkley RA: Neuropsychological and academic functioning in preschool boys with attention deficit hyperactivity disorder. Developmental Neuropsychology 13:111–129, 1997

Marshall RM, Hynd GW, Handwerk MJ, et al: Academic underachievement in ADHD subtypes. J Learn Disabil 30:635–642, 1997

Martinussen R, Frijters J, Tannock R: Naming speed and stimulant effects in attention-deficit/hyperactivity disorder. Scientific Proceedings of the American Academy of Child and Adolescent Psychiatry Meeting, Anaheim, CA, October 27–November 1, 1998

McGee R, Partridge F, Williams S, et al: A twelve year follow-up of preschool hyperactive children. J Am Acad Child Adolesc Psychiatry 30:224–232, 1991

Meyer MS, Wood FB, Hart LA, et al: Selective predictive value of rapid automatized naming in poor readers. J Learn Disabil 31:106–117, 1998

Mostofsky SH, Reiss AL, Lockhart P, et al: Evaluation of cerebellar size in attention-deficit hyperactivity disorder. J Child Neurol 13:434–439, 1998

Närhi V, Ahonen T: Reading disability with and without attention deficit hyperactivity disorder: do attentional problems make a difference? Dev Neuropsychol 11:337–350, 1995

Nicolson RI, Fawcett AJ: Comparison of deficits in cognitive and motor skills among children with dyslexia. Annals of Dyslexia 44:147–164, 1994a

Nicolson RI, Fawcett AJ: Reaction times and dyslexia. Q J Exp Psychol A 47:29–48, 1994b

Nicolson RI, Fawcett AJ, Dean P: Time estimation deficits in developmental dyslexia: evidence of cerebellar involvement. Proc R Soc Lond B Biol Sci 259:43–47, 1995

Nicolson RI, Fawcett AJ, Berry EL, et al: Association of abnormal cerebellar activation with motor learning difficulties in dyslexic adults. Lancet 353:1662–1667, 1999

Nigg JT, Hinshaw SP, Carte ET, et al: Neuropsychological correlates of childhood attention-deficit/hyperactivity disorder; explainable by comorbid disruptive behavior or reading problems? J Abnorm Psychol 107:468–480, 1998

Norrelgen F, Lacerda F, Forssberg H: Speech discrimination and phonological working memory in children with ADHD. Dev Med Child Neurol 41:335–339, 1999

Nottelmann E, Jensen P: Comorbidity of disorders in children and adolescents: developmental perspectives, in Advances in Clinical Child Psychology, Vol 17. Edited by Ollendick T, Prinz R. New York, Plenum, 1995, pp 109–155

Oosterlaan J, Logan GD, Sergeant JA: Response inhibition in AD/HD, CD, comorbid AD/HD+CD, anxious and control children: a meta-analysis of studies with the stop task. J Child Psychol Psychiatry 39:411–426, 1998

Oram J, Fine J, Tannock R: Assessing the language of children with attention deficit hyperactivity disorder. American Journal of Speech-Language Pathology 8:72–80, 1999

Ornoy A, Uriel L, Tennenbaum A: Inattention, hyperactivity and speech delay at 2-4 years of age as a predictor for ADD-ADHD syndrome. Isr J Psychiatry Relat Sci 30:155–163, 1993

Paternite CE, Loney J, Roberts MA: A preliminary validation of subtypes of DSM-IV Attention-Deficit/Hyperactivity Disorder. Journal of Attention Disorders 1:70–86, 1996

Peeke S, Halliday R, Callaway E, et al: Effects of two doses of methylphenidate on verbal information processing in hyperactive children. J Clin Psychopharmacol 4:82–88, 1984

Pelham WE Jr, Carlson C, Sams SE, et al: Separate and combined effects of methylphenidate and behavior modification on boys with attention deficit–hyperactivity disorder in the classroom. J Consult Clin Psychol 61(3):506–515, 1993

Pennington BF, Ozonoff S: Executive functions and developmental psychopathology. J Child Psychol Psychiatry 37:51–87, 1996

Pennington BF, Groisser D, Welsh MC: Contrasting cognitive deficits in attention deficit hyperactivity disorder versus reading disability. Developmental Psychology 29:511–523, 1993

Piek JP, Pitcher TM, Hay DA: Motor coordination and kinaesthesis in boys with attention-deficit hyperactivity disorder. Develop Med Child Neurol 41:159–165, 1999

Piven J, Palmer P: Cognitive deficits in parents from multiple-incidence autism families. J Child Psychol Psychiatry 38:1011–1021, 1997

Prechtl HF: Qualitative changes of spontaneous movements in fetus and preterm infant are a marker of neurological dysfunction. Early Hum Dev 23:151–158, 1990

Prechtl HF, Ferrari F, Cioni G: Predictive value of general movements in asphyxiated full-term infants. Early Hum Dev 35:91–120, 1993

Prizant BM, Audet LR, Burke GM, et al: Communication disorders and emotional/behavioral disorders in children and adolescents. Journal of Speech and Hearing Disorders 55:179–192, 1990

Purvis KL, Tannock R: Language abilities in children with attention deficit hyperactivity disorder, reading disabilities, and normal controls. J Abnorm Child Psychol 25:133–144, 1997

Purvis K, Tannock R: Contrasting cognitive abilities in children with attention deficit hyperactivity disorder and reading disability. J Am Acad Child Adolesc Psychiatry 39:4, 2000

Rae C, Lee MA, Dixon RM, et al: Metabolic abnormalities in developmental dyslexia detected by 1H magnetic resonance spectroscopy. Lancet 351:1849–1852, 1998

Rasmussen P, Gillberg C: Chapter, in A Neurodevelopmental Approach to Specific Learning Disorders: Clinics in Developmental Medicine, Vol 145. Edited by Whitmore K, Hart H, Willems G. Oxford, UK, MacKeith Press, 1999, pp 134–156

Rasmussen P, Gillberg C, Waldenstrom E, et al: Perceptual, motor and attentional deficits in seven-year-old children: neurological and neurodevelopmental aspects. Dev Med Child Neurol 25:315–333, 1983

Reader MJ, Harris EL, Schuerholz LJ, et al: Attention deficit hyperactivity disorder and executive dysfunction. Developmental Neuropsychology 10:493–512, 1994

Richardson E, Kupietz SS, Winsberg BG, et al: Effects of methylphenidate dosage in hyperactive reading-disabled children, II: reading achievement. J Am Acad Child Adolesc Psychiatry 27:78–87, 1988

Rispens J, van Yperen TA: How specific are "specific developmental disorders"? the relevance of the concept of specific developmental disorders for the classification of childhood developmental disorders. J Child Psychol Psychiatry 38:351–363, 1997

Rubia K, Overmeyer S, Taylor E, et al: Hypofrontality in attention deficit hyperactivity disorder during higher-order motor control: a study with functional MRI. Am J Psychiatry 156:891–896, 1999

Rutter M: Comorbidity: meanings and mechanisms. Clinical Psychology; Science and Practice 1:100–103, 1994

Rutter M, Lord C: Language disorders associated with psychiatric disturbance, in Language Development and Disorders. Edited by Yule W, Rutter M. Oxford, England, McKeith Press, 1987, pp 206–233

Saltzman EL, Munhall KG: A dynamical approach to gestural patterning in speech production. Ecological Psychology 1:333–382, 1989

Schachar RJ: Hyperkinetic syndrome: historical development of the concept, in The Overactive Child. Edited by Taylor EA. Philadelphia, PA, JB Lippincott, 1986, pp 19–40

Schmahmann JD, Sherman JC: The cerebellar cognitive affective syndrome. Brain 121:561–579, 1998

Schuerholz LJ, Harris EL, Baumgardner TL, et al: An analysis of two discrepancy-based models and a processing-deficit approach in identifying learning disabilities. J Learn Disabil 28:18–29, 1995

Semrud-Clikeman M, Sprich-Buckminster S, Krifcher Lehman B, et al: Comorbidity between ADDH and learning disability: a review and report in a clinically referred sample. J Am Acad Child Adolesc Psychiatry 31:439–448, 1992

Shaywitz BA, Shaywitz SE: Comorbidity: a critical issue in attention deficit disorder. J Child Neurol 6 (suppl):S13–S22, 1991

Shaywitz B, Fletcher J, Shaywitz S: Defining and classifying learning disabilities and attention-deficit/hyperactivity disorder. J Child Neurol 10 (suppl):S50–S57, 1995

Shaywitz SE, Shaywitz BA, Fletcher JM, et al: Prevalence of reading disability in boys and girls: results of the Connecticut Longitudinal Study. JAMA 264:998–1002, 1990

Shaywitz SE, Fletcher JM, Shaywitz BA: A conceptual model and definition of dyslexia: findings emerging from the Connecticut Longitudinal Study, in Language, Learning, and Behavior Disorders: Developmental, Biological, and Clinical Perspectives. Edited by Beitchman JH, Cohen N, Konstantareas MM, et al. New York, Cambridge University, 1996, pp 199–223

Smith SD, Pennington B, Fulker DW, et al: Evidence for a gene influencing reading disability on chromosome 6p in two populations. Am J Hum Genet 55:A203, 1994

Stein JF, Glickstein M: Role of the cerebellum in the visual guidance of movement. Physiol Rev 72:967–1017, 1992

Stein J, Walsh V: To see but not to read: the magnocellular theory of dyslexia. Trends Neurosci 20:147–152, 1997

Stevenson J: Developmental changes in the mechanisms linking language disabilities and behavior disorders, in Language, Learning and Behaviour Disorders: Developmental, Biological, and Clinical Perspectives. Edited by Beitchman JH, Cohen N, Konstantareas MM, et al. Cambridge, UK, Cambridge University Press, 1996, pp 78–99

Stevenson J, Pennington BF, Gilger JW, et al: Hyperactivity and spelling disability: testing for shared genetic aetiology. J Child Psychol Psychiatry 34:1137–1152, 1993

Swanson JM, Sunohara GA, Kennedy JL, et al: Association of the dopamine receptor D4 (DRD4) gene with a refined phenotype of attention deficit hyperactivity disorder (ADHD): a family-based approach. Mol Psychiatry 3:38–41, 1998

Szatmari P, Offord D, Boyle MH: Correlates, associated impairments, and patterns of service utilization of children with attention deficit disorders: findings from the Ontario Child Health Study. J Child Psychol Psychiatry 30:205–217, 1989a

Szatmari P, Offord DR, Boyle MH: Ontario Child Health Study: prevalence of attention deficit disorder with hyperactivity. J Child Psychol Psychiatry 30:219–230, 1989b

Tallal P, Ross R, Curtiss S: Familial aggregation in specific language impairment. Journal of Speech and Hearing Disorders 54:167–173, 1989

Tannock R: Attention deficit hyperactivity disorder: advances in cognitive, neurobiological, and genetic research. J Child Psychol Psychiatry 39:65–99, 1998

Tannock R: Methylphenidate: Effects on language, reading, and auditory processing, in Ritalin: Theory and Practice, 2nd Edition. Edited by Greenhill LL, Osman B. Larchmont, NY, Mary Ann Liebert, 1999, pp 265–285

Tannock R: Time perception, inhibition and stimulant effects. Paper presented at the 10th annual Eunethydis Meeting: Image Project and Neurobiopsychology of Hyperkinesis. Paris, France, November 20–21, 1999

Tannock R: Cognitive correlates of attention deficit hyperactivity disorder, in Diagnosis and Treatment of Attention Deficit Hyperactivity Disorder: An Evidence-Based Approach. Edited by Jensen P, Cooper J. New York, American Medical Association Press (in press)

Tannock R, Schachar R: Executive dysfunction as an underlying mechanism of behavior and language problems in attention deficit hyperactivity disorder, in Language, Learning and Behaviour Disorders: Developmental, Biological, and Clinical Perspectives. Edited by Beitchman JH, Cohen N, Konstantareas MM, et al. Cambridge, UK, Cambridge University Press, 1996, pp 128–155

Tannock R, Purvis K, Schachar R: Narrative abilities in children with attention deficit hyperactivity disorder and normal peers. J Abnorm Child Psychol 21:103–117, 1993

Thach WT: On the specific role of the cerebellum in motor learning and cognition: clues from PET activation and lesion studies in man, in Motor Learning and Synaptic Plasticity in the Cerebellum. Edited by Cordo PJ, Bell CC, Harnad S. New York, Cambridge University Press, 1997, pp 73–93

Tirosh E, Cohen A: Language deficit with attention-deficit disorder: a prevalent comorbidity. J Child Neurol 13:493–497, 1998

Tripp G, Luk SL, Schaughency EA, et al: DSM-IV and ICD-10: a comparison of the correlates of ADHD and hyperkinetic disorder. J Am Acad Child Adolesc Psychiatry 38:156–164, 1999

Van der Meere JJ: The role of attention, in Hyperactivity Disorders of Childhood. Edited by Sandberg S. Cambridge, UK, Cambridge University Press, 1996, pp 111–148

Vandervelden MC, Siegel LS: Phonological recoding deficits and dyslexia: a developmental perspective, in Language, Learning, and Behavior Disorders: Developmental, Biological, and Clinical Perspectives. Edited by Beitchman JH, Cohen N, Konstantareas MM, et al. New York, Cambridge University Press, 1996, pp 224–226

Wagner RK, Torgeson JK, Rashott CA: Development of reading-related phonological processing abilities: new evidence of bidirectional causality from a latent variable longitudinal study. Developmental Psychology 30:73–87, 1994

Weiss G, Hechtman LT: Hyperactive Children Grown Up: ADHD in Children, Adolescents, and Adults. New York, Guilford, 1993

Whalen CK, Henker B, Collins BE, et al: Peer interaction in a structured communication task: comparisons of normal and hyperactive boys and of methylphenidate (Ritalin) and placebo effects. Child Dev 50:388–401, 1979

Whitmont S, Clark C: Kinaesthetic acuity and fine motor skills in children with attention deficit hyperactivity disorder: a preliminary report. Dev Med Child Neurol 38:1091–1098, 1996

Whitmore K, Bax M: Checking the health of school entrants. Archives of Diseases of Childhood 65:320–326, 1990

Wilson P, McKenzie B: Information processing deficits associated with developmental coordination disorder: a meta-analysis of research findings. J Child Psychol Psychiatry 39:829–840, 1998

Wimmer H: Characteristics of developmental dyslexia in a regular writing system. Applied Psycholinguistics 14:1–34, 1993

Wolf M: Naming speed and reading: the contribution of the cognitive neurosciences. Reading Research Quarterly 26:123–141, 1991

Wolff PH, Melngailis I: Family patterns of developmental dyslexia: clinical findings. Am J Med Genet 54:122–131, 1994

Wolff PH, Michel GF, Ovrut M, et al: Rate and timing precision of motor co-ordination in developmental dyslexia. Dev Psychol 26:349–359, 1990

Wolff PH, Melngailis I, Obregon M, et al: Family patterns of developmental dyslexia, part II: behavioral phenotypes. Am J Med Genet 60:494–505, 1995

Wolff PH, Melngailis I, Kotwica K: Family patterns of developmental dyslexia, part III: spelling errors as behavioral phenotype. Am J Med Genet 67:378–386, 1996

Wolraich ML, Hannah JN, Pinnock TY, et al: Comparison of diagnostic criteria for attention-deficit hyperactivity disorder in a country-wide sample. J Am Acad Child Adolesc Psychiatry 35:319–324, 1996

World Health Organization: International Statistical Classification of Diseases and Related Health Problems, 10th Revision. Geneva, World Health Organization, 1992

Zentall SS: Production deficiencies in elicited language but not in the spontaneous verbalizations of hyperactive children. J Abnorm Child Psychol 16:657–673, 1988

Zentall SS, Gohs DE, Culatta B: Language and activity of hyperactive and comparison children during listening tasks. Exceptional Children 50:255–266, 1983

Afterword

Laurence L. Greenhill, M.D.

The five chapters in this text provide a timely overview of the field of learning disabilities. This field is of crucial importance for professionals of all backgrounds because learning disabilities affect so many domains of both child and adult functioning, causing problems in many areas of living and adaptation. Learning disabilities afflict both children and adults and cause frustration, demoralization, poor self-esteem, and difficulties in everyday life. It behooves the professional to have a better understanding of the field.

I hope that the information in these chapters not only provides practical guidance for psychiatrists and psychologists but also serves as an introduction to one of the most important areas for patients and their diagnoses. In closing, I wish to thank the contributors to this text for providing a superb, scholarly, and informative introduction to this most exciting field.

Index

*Page numbers printed in **boldface** type refer to tables or figures.*

Diagnosis. *See also* Assessment;
    Evaluation
    of ADHD, 98
    of depression in children, 48
    of dyslexia, 79–84
    follow-up study of
        uncomplicated reading
        disorder and, 14
    of learning disorders and
        comorbid psychiatric
        disorders, 40–41
Diagnostic Interview Schedule
    for Children (DISC-IV), 98,
    104, 105, 110
Dimensional model, of dyslexia, 60
Discrepancy approach, to
    diagnosis of learning
    disorders
    controversy on, 99–100
    dyslexia and, 81
    specific learning disabilities
        (SLD) and, 104
    study of comorbid ADHD and
        learning disabilities and,
        111–123
Domain-specific assessment, of
    learning disorders, 36–37
DSM-II, and hyperkinetic
    reaction to childhood, 100
DSM-III
    ADHD and, 100, 101
    conduct disorder and, 3–4
DSM-III-R, and ADHD, 100, 101
DSM-IV
    ADHD and, 84, 97, 100, 101,
        110, 122, 129–131, 138, 142
    classification of learning
        disorders in, 38–39
    communication disorders and
        motor skills disorders in,
        129–131

definition of learning
    disorders in, 1, 36
depression in children and, 48
simple difference method for
    evaluation of learning
    disorders and, 112
Dyslexia
    cerebellar dysfunction and,
        149
    cognitive basis of, 61–63,
        87–88
    diagnosis and evaluation of,
        79–84
    epidemiology of, 60–61
    genetics and, 150
    management of, 84–87
    neural basis for, 63–79
    oral language skills and, 39
    prevalence of, 59, 60
Dysthymia, 47, 48

Echo planar imaging, and
    dyslexia, 68
Educational attainment, and
    uncomplicated reading
    disorder, 17, **18,** 25
Education for All Handicapped
    Children Act (1975), 35, 102
Educational services, and
    guidelines for ADHD,
    100–104. *See also* Schools;
    Special education
Employment history, and follow-
    up study of uncomplicated
    reading disorder, 25–26. *See
    also* Occupational status
Epidemiology. *See also* Prevalence
    of dyslexia, 60–61
    of learning disorders, 39–40
Etiology, of learning disorders,
    37, 146–151

Phonological processing
   ADHD and, 139–140
   brain activation patterns and,
      71–72, **73**
   dyslexia and, 71, 87, 88
   reading disorder and, 136
Positron-emission tomography
   (PET) studies
   of cerebellar role in timing,
      148
   of dyslexia, 66–67, 149
Posterior parietal cortex, and
   dyslexia, 150
Pragmatic language disorders,
   and ADHD, 134–135,
   136–137
Predicted achievement method,
   for assessment of learning
   disorders, 99, 101–102, 112,
   113, 114, 115, **118–119,** 120,
   122, 123
Prefrontal cortex, and ADHD,
   148, 151
Prevalence. *See also*
   Epidemiology
   of dyslexia, 59, 60
   of learning disorders and
      comorbid ADHD, 3,
      43–45, 51, 98, 132–133,
      134, 135–136, 142
   of learning disorders and
      comorbid psychiatric
      disorders, 33, 34
   of reading disorders, 1–2, 39
Probable diagnosis, 14
Processing disorders, federal
   regulations and definition of,
   35–36
Pronunciation tasks, and brain
   imaging studies of dyslexia,
   65, 67

Psychiatric status, and
   uncomplicated reading
   disorder, 14–15, 20–23
Psychometric tests, and
   assessment of learning
   disorders, 98–99, 110
Psychostimulants. *See* Stimulants
Psychotherapy, for comorbid
   learning disabilities and
   psychiatric disorders, 51
Public health, and reading
   disorders, 2

Quantity, of language and
   ADHD, 136–137

Rapid automatized naming, and
   spina bifida, 140
Reading. *See also* Reading
   disorders
   functional magnetic resonance
      imaging (fMRI) studies of
      dyslexia and, **65,** 68–79
   learning disorders presenting
      with difficulties of, **85**
Reading disorders. *See also*
   Reading; Uncomplicated
   reading disorder
   ADHD and, 137–141, 145–146,
      151–152
   behavioral problems and,
      2–4
   cerebellar dysfunction and,
      149–150
   DSM-IV criteria for, 38
   emotional and behavioral
      adjustment and, 2
   gender and, 39
   prevalence of, 1–2
   relative stability of through
      childhood, 2

Reading disorders. *See also*
Reading; Uncomplicated
reading disorder *(continued)*
review of longitudinal and
follow-up studies on,
4–8
stimulants and, 145–146
Receptive language disorders,
134–136
Rehabilitation Act of 1973, 103
Remediation programs, for
reading and ADHD, 152
Right cerebellar cortex, and
dyslexia, 149
Right hemisphere, of brain. *See
also* Hemispheres of brain
dyslexia and, 74–75
gender and phonological
processing, **72**
nonverbal learning disabilities
and, 44

Scales of Independent Behavior
(SIB), 114
School-age children, and
diagnosis of dyslexia, **83**
School refusal, 13
Schools. *See also* Educational
services; Special education;
Teachers
dyslexia and management in,
86
reading disorders and
behavioral problems in, 3
social skills and, 42
treatment of comorbid
learning disabilities and
psychiatric disorders and,
52
Selective attention, and learning
disabilities, 44–45

Self-esteem
learning disabilities and, 42, 43
reading disorders and, 4, 26
Sensory deficits
dyslexia and, 84
reading disorders and, 38
Separation anxiety disorder, 9, 13
SES (socioeconomic status), and
reading disorders, 12, 13, **16,**
17
Side effects, of stimulant
medications, 51
Significant discrepancy, and
discrepancy method for
assessment of learning
disorders, 99, 115, 120, 122,
123
Simple difference method, for
assessment of learning
disorders, 99, 112, 113,
118–119, 120
SLD. *See* Specific Learning
Disabilities
SNAP-IV (Swanson, Nolan, and
Pelham) rating scale, 98,
104–105, **106–107, 109,** 110,
121
Social-emotional development,
and learning disorders,
41–43
Social functioning and social
skills
follow-up study of
uncomplicated reading
disorder and, 23
nonverbal learning disabilities
and, 40
schools and development of, 42
Socioeconomic status (SES), and
reading disorders, 12, 13, **16,**
17